Contents

Preface

The days when type 2 diabetes was labelled a "mild" form of the condition are long gone. Recent years have demonstrated dramatically that diabetes is a major public health issue not just because of the sheer numbers of sufferers, but also because of the long-term complications, principally cardiovascular disease, which will kill around 80% of type 2 diabetic patients – many prematurely.

Over the past 20 years clinicians have recognized that type 2 diabetes is part of a syndrome of chronic cardiovascular risk, but we have only recently had an unequivocal evidence base for management.

It has been a great pleasure to write this book for the primary care multi-professional team because "diabetes and the heart" has become one of the biggest public health issues of our time. We have attempted to define precisely what the problem is, emphasizing the scale, aetiology, diagnosis and treatment. We have discussed the relationship between the major cardiovascular risk factors and the enormous evidence base we now have for treatment. This includes the importance of lifestyle intervention, such as weight loss, physical activity and smoking cessation, and aggressive screening for and management of glycaemia, lipids and blood pressure.

We now have evidence for treatment and the drugs to do the job (although even better drugs will undoubtedly be developed in the future), but the real challenge is putting it into practice and overcoming patient compliance and concordance problems. We have therefore tried to provide a highly practical approach to management, illustrated with case studies. The book also contains a comprehensive list of relevant drugs, with information on doses, efficacy and side-effects, and we have referenced the book thoroughly throughout.

There is no doubt that to make an impact on the terrible rates of attrition from diabetes we must focus on cardiovascular disease. We hope you will find this book interesting and informative and that it will help your approach to clinical practice in this important area.

Anthony Barnett
Professor of Medicine and Consultant Physician
University of Birmingham and
Birmingham Heartlands Hospital
Birmingham, UK

Geraldine O'Gara
General Practitioner and Hospital Practitioner in Diabetes
East Birmingham Primary Care Trust and
Birmingham Heartlands Hospital
Birmingham, UK

Biographies

Anthony H Barnett MBBS, BSc (Hons), MD, FRCP is Professor of Medicine, University of Birmingham, and Consultant Physician and Head of Diabetes Services, Birmingham Heartlands and Solihull NHS Trust (Teaching).

Professor Barnett has published over 300 papers on the genetics of diabetes and microangiopathic complications, genetics of other autoimmune diseases and on many aspects of diabetic vascular disease. He also has a major clinical (as well as research) interest in diabetes and vascular disease. He runs one of the largest diabetic clinics in the country. He has lectured extensively in his areas of interest.

He has also edited and contributed to many major books in diabetes and vascular disease, including editing Hypertension and Diabetes (now in its third edition), Diabetes, Lipids and Vascular Disease (now in its second edition) and Shared Care in Diabetes. He is also editor of four quarterly educational journals aimed at primary care – Modern Diabetes Management, Modern Hypertension Management, Obesity in Practice and Practical Cardiovascular Risk Management. He has contributed to Textbook of Diabetes, International Textbook of Diabetes and the Encyclopaedia of Molecular Biology and Biotechnology.

Geraldine O'Gara MBBCh, BAO, MRCGP has worked as a GP in Small Heath, Birmingham for 20 years. She has had a special interest in diabetes since her GP registrar days in east London when her "project" was to set up the diabetes clinic in the practice. She works for two sessions a week in the local hospital diabetic clinic.

Introduction

The first description of diabetes mellitus was in the ancient Egyptian writings, the Ebers Papyrus, some three-and-a-half thousand years ago. The Egyptians thought diabetes was due to an "imbalance of the four bodily elements" and the treatment was a mixture of ground earth, water, wheat and lead! Treatments have improved since then, but we still have a long way to go in applying current knowledge and evidence to the benefit of diabetic patients.

66 We have a long way to go in applying current evidence to the benefit of diabetic patients 99

Diabetes is a major public health problem world-wide. Around 200 million people have the condition, and this is predicted to increase to 300 million by 2020.[1] In the UK alone, the number of diabetic patients is approaching 2 million and this is estimated to rise to 3 million by 2010 (Figure 1). The vast majority have type 2 diabetes. The exponential rise in numbers is due in part to the ageing population, but also to the explosion in obesity rates in many parts of the world as a result of overnutrition and inactivity. Although the problem of type 1 diabetes must not be ignored, it is dwarfed by the sheer numbers of patients with type 2 diabetes.

Diabetes is a devastating disease because of its long-term vascular complications, which are:
* Cardiovascular
  - coronary heart disease
  - stroke
  - peripheral vascular disease
* Microvascular involving
  - eyes
  - kidneys
  - peripheral nerves.

66 Around 80% of all diabetic patients will die from cardiovascular complications 99

The consequences[2,3] are that:
* around 80% of all diabetic patients will die, many prematurely, from cardiovascular complications, particularly coronary heart disease
* diabetic eye disease is the commonest cause of blindness in the working population in western Europe and the US
* diabetic kidney disease is the single most common reason for chronic renal failure and the need for dialysis
* diabetic foot problems are the commonest reason for non-traumatic lower limb amputation in western Europe and the US.

The costs of diabetes are high and are increasing.[4,5] In the UK diabetes consumes around 9% of the total healthcare budget with 80% of costs related to the long-term complications. In the US the figures are even worse – around 15% of the total healthcare budget is spent on diabetes and its complications. These are the costs to the Exchequer, but add to this the personal costs to the patient and their family and

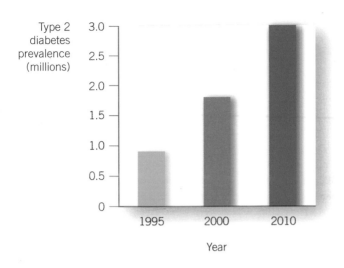

Fig. 1. Prevalence of type 2 diabetes in the UK with projections to the year 2010. Adapted from Diabet Med 1997;14 (Suppl 5): 57-85 with permission from Blackwell Publishing.

one can imagine this condition is one of the most important healthcare challenges we face.

That was the bad news! On the positive side, a range of treatments has been developed for managing diabetes and its complications, and over the last decade or so many major studies have provided an excellent evidence base from which to manage the disease. This is particularly the case for cardiovascular risk factor intervention. Studies have unequivocally shown dramatic reductions in cardiovascular end points and mortality by appropriate treatments. The challenge is putting the evidence into practice given the massive and increasing numbers of patients and the wide range of complications from which they suffer.

Unfortunately, the general public and some healthcare professionals still think of type 2 diabetes as the "mild" form of the condition. Nothing could be further from the truth. Indeed, the risk that a diabetic patient, or even a patient in the pre-diabetic phase, will suffer a cardiovascular event or death is vastly magnified compared with the general population. We do our patients a grave disservice when we tell them they have "a touch of diabetes" and that it is nothing to worry about.

66 Studies have shown dramatic reductions in mortality by appropriate treatments 99

Definition and epidemiology

Diabetes has been defined as "a state of premature cardiovascular death that is associated with chronic hyperglycaemia and may also be associated with blindness and renal failure".[6] The point is that diabetes is a cardiovascular disease, and we should therefore not focus on blood glucose alone. Cardiovascular or macrovascular disease is easily the

Fig. 2. Patients with type 2 diabetes without previous myocardial infarction have as high a risk of myocardial infarction as non-diabetic patients with previous myocardial infarction.

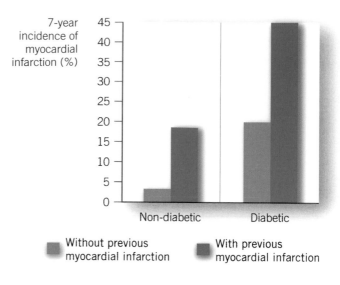

Without previous myocardial infarction

With previous myocardial infarction

> Cardiovascular disease is easily the greatest cause of morbidity and premature death in diabetic patients

> More than 50% of diabetic patients have evidence of cardiovascular disease at diagnosis

greatest cause of morbidity and premature death in diabetic patients (Figure 2).[7-9]

- Patients with diabetes have twice the risk of coronary heart disease compared with the general population.
- More than 50% of diabetic patients have evidence of cardiovascular disease at diagnosis.
- Men with diabetes and no history of myocardial infarction have the same chance of a coronary event as men without diabetes who have previously had such an event.[10]
- The increased risk of cardiovascular mortality is even greater in women.[11]
- Atherosclerotic disease involving the coronary (Figure 3), cerebral (Figure 4) and peripheral blood vessels (Figures 5 and 6) occurs at an earlier age and with greater frequency in diabetic patients.[12]
- Although patients with diabetes account for only 3% to 5% of the population, they represent 10% to 15% of those admitted to hospital with myocardial infarction and up to 20% of those who die.[13]
- Coronary heart disease tends to be more severe than in non-diabetic people with cardiovascular disease, and is associated with poorer outcomes.[13] The reasons for this include development of heart disease at a younger age, involvement of more coronary vessels and increased likelihood of congestive heart failure.
- Outcomes following myocardial infarction are worse than in non-diabetic people with increased rates of heart failure and death in both the early post-infarction period and for several years after the event.[13]

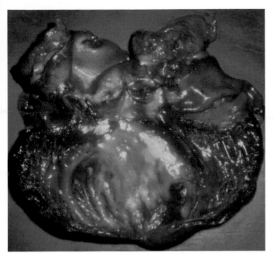

Fig. 3. Post-mortem specimen of a heart showing massive myocardial infarction causing death of a diabetic patient.

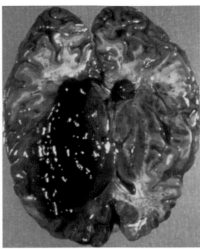

Fig. 4. Post-mortem specimen of the brain of a diabetic patient who died of a cerebrovascular accident.

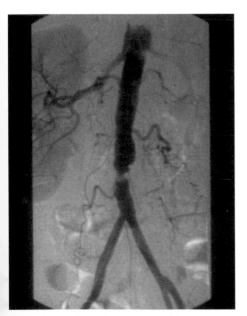

Fig. 5. Arteriogram of the peripheral vasculature of a diabetic patient showing arterial narrowing.
Published with grateful thanks to Dr John Henderson, Consultant Radiologist.

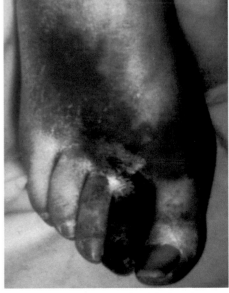

Fig. 6. Gangrene of the foot of a diabetic patient with spreading infection requiring below knee amputation.

9

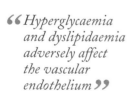
These facts suggest the concept of primary prevention of cardiovascular disease in diabetic patients is redundant. Strategies for managing type 2 diabetes must be similar or identical to those used for established cardiovascular disease.

Aetiology

The essential lesion in both type 1 and type 2 diabetes is accelerated atherosclerosis (Figure 7), with alterations in endothelial cell and platelet interactions and abnormalities in lipid and lipoprotein metabolism (Figures 8 and 9).[14] Hyperglycaemia *per se* adversely affects vascular endothelium, and this in part explains the increased risk of cardiovascular disease in type 1 diabetes.

The problem of cardiovascular disease is greatly compounded in type 2 diabetes because of the common co-occurrence of cardiovascular risk factors. Hyperglycaemia and dyslipidaemia adversely affect the vascular endothelium. Hypertension increases the risk of vascular endothelial injury with subsequent macrophage and platelet aggregation, the release of growth factors that stimulate

66 Hyperglycaemia and dyslipidaemia adversely affect the vascular endothelium 99

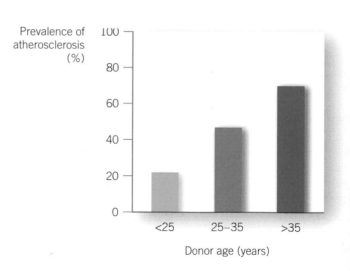

Fig. 7. Atherosclerosis (determined by coronary intravascular ultrasound) starts at a young age. This effect is magnified in people with diabetes. Data is taken from post-mortem specimens from people who died as a result of accidents etc. Reprinted from Nissen S. Coronary angiography and intravascular ultrasound. Am J Cardiol 2001;87(suppl):15A-20 with permission from Excerpta Medica, Inc.

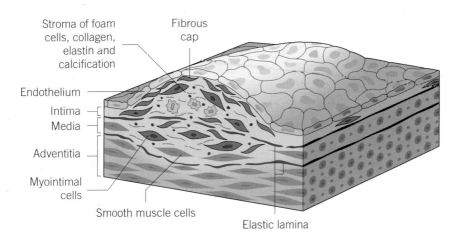

Stroma of foam cells, collagen, elastin and calcification

Fibrous cap

Endothelium

Intima

Media

Adventitia

Myointimal cells

Smooth muscle cells

Elastic lamina

Fig. 8. Diagramatic representation of a cross section of a fibrous plaque, the hallmark of established atherosclerosis. Reproduced with permission from Lipids, Diabetes and Vascular Disease (second edition). Dodson PM, Barnett AH (eds). London: Science Press Ltd. 1998; p1.

proliferation of smooth muscle cells and deposition of lipid-laden foam cells.

Syndrome of chronic cardiovascular risk

Cardiovascular risk factors commonly co-occur in the same patient at a frequency much higher than expected by chance. This is postulated to relate to the primary underlying abnormality of insulin resistance (resistance of the body to the biological actions of insulin) (Figure 10).[15] The major arbiters of insulin resistance are obesity and sedentary lifestyle, although genetic factors are also involved. Around 25% of the adult UK population are now insulin resistant coincident with the massive increase in obesity rates seen in this country and elsewhere.[16,17]

66 25% of the adult UK population are insulin resistant 99

The consequences of insulin resistance include:
- Increased insulin secretion from the pancreas (hyperinsulinaemia)
- Hyperinsulinaemia is associated with a dyslipidaemic, atherogenic lipid profile with increases in low- and very-low-density lipoproteins (LDL and VLDL) and a reduction in the anti-atherogenic high-density lipoprotein (HDL).[18]
- Insulin resistance and hyperinsulinaemia are also associated with development of hypertension, perhaps through increased sodium

Fig. 9. Postulated biochemical processes involved in the accelerated atherosclerosis of diabetes.
Reproduced with permission from Lipids, Diabetes and Vascular disease (second edition). Dodson PM, Barnett AH (eds). London: Science Press Ltd, 1998; p27

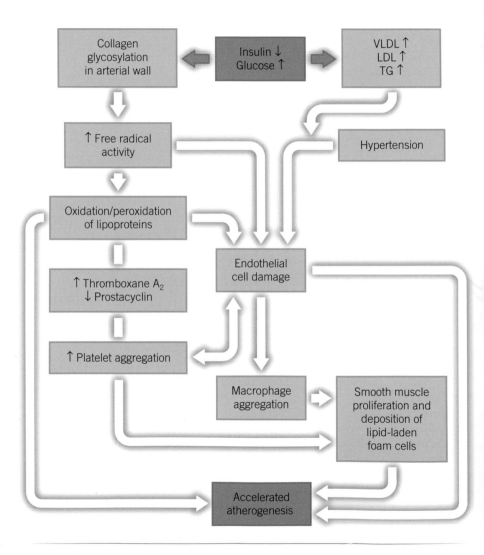

LDL = low-density lipoprotein; VLDL = very-low-density lipoprotein; TG = triglycerides

re-absorption from the proximal renal tubules of the kidney and increased sympathetic nervous system stimulation.[19,20]

- Not all insulin-resistant people will develop glucose intolerance, but in a significant proportion the pancreas will eventually secrete insufficient insulin to overcome the insulin resistance, leading initially to impaired glucose tolerance followed by frank type 2 diabetes.

This concept of a syndrome of chronic cardiovascular risk (also called insulin resistance or metabolic syndrome) has been one of the most important developments in our understanding and practical management of type 2 diabetes. Since the original description in 1988,[15] other abnormalities have been added to the syndrome, including microalbuminuria (renal protein leakage above the normal range but

> **❝Age-related mortality increases significantly with increasing BMI❞**

Fig. 10. Metabolic syndrome hypothesis. This relates the common co-occurrence of cardiovascular risk factors in the same patient to insulin resistance.

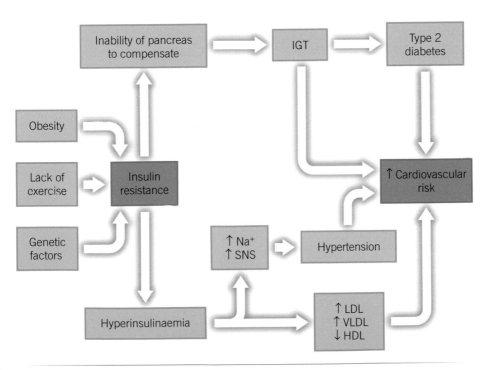

IGT = impaired glucose tolerance; ↑Na⁺ = increased sodium reabsorption from the kidney; ↑SNS = increased sympathetic nervous system stimulation; LDL, VLDL, HDL = low-, very-low, high-density lipoprotein

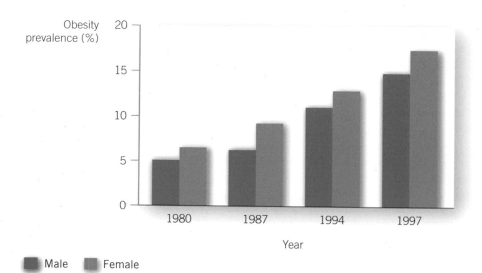

Obesity prevalence (%)

Year

■ Male   ■ Female

Fig. 11. Prevalence of obesity in England since 1980. Prevalence is now around 20% in both sexes.

below the level of dipstick testing), clotting abnormalities and increased inflammatory markers.

Putting all this together, there is clearly a strong relationship between the lifestyle changes that have occurred in many parts of the world in the past few decades and development of insulin resistance, type 2 diabetes and other major cardiovascular risk factors.

Obesity, type 2 diabetes and cardiovascular risk

Obesity, defined as a body mass index (BMI) over 30kg/m², now affects around 20% of the UK adult population (Figure 11) and over 30% of the US population, and around two thirds of both populations are overweight or obese.[16,17] Age-related mortality increases significantly with increasing BMI, and even at a BMI over 27kg/m² around

Fig. 12. Obesity and its relationship to cardiovascular disease and death: the Framingham study.[8] Results were independent of age, cholesterol, blood pressure, glucose tolerance, smoking or left ventricular hypertrophy.

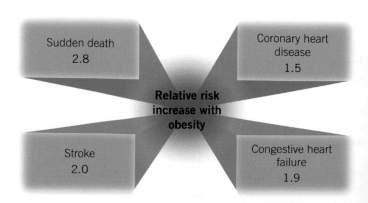

Sudden death
2.8

Coronary heart disease
1.5

Relative risk increase with obesity

Stroke
2.0

Congestive heart failure
1.9

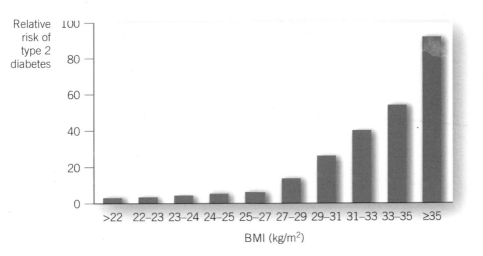

Relative risk of type 2 diabetes / BMI (kg/m²)

Fig. 13. Relative risk of type 2 diabetes with increasing BMI.

75% of people will have some evidence of a co-morbidity such as cardiovascular disease, hypertension, dyslipidaemia or type 2 diabetes.[21] This is even more of a problem in certain racial groups and has led to a recommendation from the World Health Organization (WHO) to redefine obesity in people of Asian extraction as a BMI over 25kg/m², and overweight as a BMI over 23kg/m².[22]

The Framingham study clearly showed that obesity is a significant risk factor for cardiovascular disease and death irrespective of age, blood pressure, smoking, cholesterol, family history or glucose intolerance (Figure 12).[8]

The increasing prevalence of obesity relates in part to dietary factors, particularly high-fat content. Fat is calorie dense and less appetite suppressing than carbohydrate. Even more important is sedentary lifestyle. This problem is becoming particularly marked in children where obesity rates are approximately 20% in teenagers.[23]

An even better predictor of outcomes appears to be the degree of intra-abdominal fat. So called "apple-shaped" distribution of fat or "big belly" obesity is an ominous finding and associated with dramatically increased risk of both type 2 diabetes and cardiovascular disease.[24,25] Intra-abdominal fat is metabolically active and specifically relates to development of insulin resistance. Increased visceral adiposity may be a particular issue in people of Indo-Asian extraction who tend to have a high waist/hip ratio and increased cardiovascular and diabetes risk.[26]

Obesity is the single most important reason for the vast increase in rates of type 2 diabetes worldwide (Figure 13). It is the most important modifiable factor for diabetes and the incidence of type 2 diabetes

❝ So called apple-shaped distribution of fat is associated with dramatically increased risk of type 2 diabetes and cardiovascular disease ❞

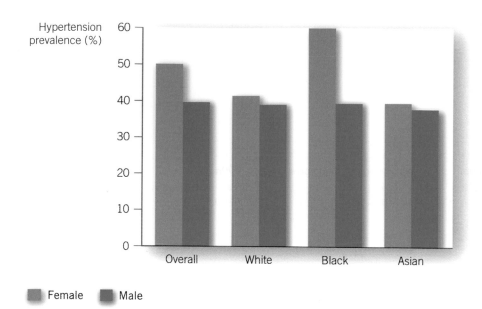

Hypertension prevalence (%)

Female   Male

Fig. 14. Prevalence of hypertension in diabetic patients from different racial groups based on old WHO criteria (blood pressure ≥160/95mmHg). Reproduced from Pacy PJ. Prevalence of hypertension in white, black and Asian diabetics in a district hospital diabetic clinic. Diabetic Med 1985;2:125-130 with permission from Blackwell Publishing.

rises with increasing severity of obesity but also with weight-gain itself, independent of baseline BMI.[27]

Diabetes and dyslipidaemia

For a given total cholesterol, the risk of coronary heart disease in diabetes is considerably magnified

The typical diabetic dyslipidaemia includes increased LDL and VLDL and reduced HDL (in practice raised triglycerides and low HDL). This profile is characteristically associated with insulin resistance and hyperinsulinaemia.[15]

The exact mechanism is unclear. Studies have shown that production of VLDL is increased in obese patients, perhaps related to increased turnover of non-esterified fatty acids, which stimulates the liver to synthesize more trigylceride-enriched VLDL, the consequence being hypertriglyceridaemia.[28] Increased circulating VLDL will lead to increased exchange of VLDL triglycerides for cholesterol esters derived from HDL and LDL. This results in reduced HDL cholesterol concentration and formation of small dense atherogenic LDL particles.

In addition, although total cholesterol may be no higher than in the non-diabetic population, there is a clear relationship between total cholesterol and coronary heart disease mortality in diabetic men parallel with, but with a four-fold greater risk than, that in men without diabetes.[7] For a given total cholesterol, the risk of coronary heart disease in diabetes is considerably magnified compared with the non-diabetic population.

Diabetes and hypertension

Based on the old WHO criteria, which defined hypertension as a blood pressure of 160/95mmHg or higher, 40% to 50% of type 2 diabetic patients would be classified as hypertensive (Figure 14). With the redefinition of hypertension as a blood pressure of 140/90mmHg or higher,[29] around 80% of patients with type 2 diabetes are now classified as hypertensive. The reason for this extremely high prevalence is not entirely clear, but may relate to insulin resistance, hyperinsulinaemia and its consequences. Obesity is clearly a major arbiter of this association as well as weight gain. Central obesity, in particular, is a powerful predictor of hypertension.

❝ 80% of patients with type 2 diabetes are now classified as hypertensive ❞

Diabetes and other cardiovascular risk factors

Cigarette smoking is a major risk factor for cardiovascular disease in both diabetic and non-diabetic people (Figure 15).

Diabetes is a prothrombotic state[28] resulting in:

increased blood viscosity

reduced blood flow in the microcirculation

several defects of coagulation and fibrinolysis.

Surrogate markers for cardiovascular risk include increased fibrinogen and plasminogen activator inhibitor 1 (PAI-1) activity, well described in diabetic patients.

The presence of protein leakage from the kidneys, defined in its earliest stages as microalbuminuria (an albumin excretion rate above the

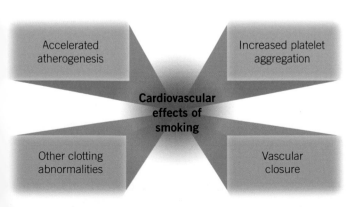

Fig. 15. Examples of how cigarette smoking contributes to cardiovascular disease.

Accelerated atherogenesis

Increased platelet aggregation

Cardiovascular effects of smoking

Other clotting abnormalities

Vascular closure

> *Microalbuminuria is a marker for leaky, damaged blood vessels*

normal range but below the level of dipstick testing), is predictive of later overt nephropathy, renal failure and, in particular, cardiovascular disease and mortality (Figures 16 and 17).[30] Microalbuminuria is a marker for "leaky", damaged blood vessels and even in non-diabetic people is associated with increased cardiovascular risk and mortality. It may be a marker for endothelial cell injury that initiates the atheromatous process.

Congestive heart failure

This is more common in diabetic patients and may account, at least in part, for the higher morbidity and mortality seen after myocardial infarction compared with the general population. Obesity itself is related to changes in cardiac structure and function with increased blood volume and cardiac output leading to left ventricular dilatation

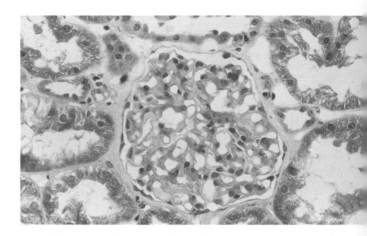

Fig. 16. Haematoxylin and eosin stain of renal glomerulus showing normal histological architecture.

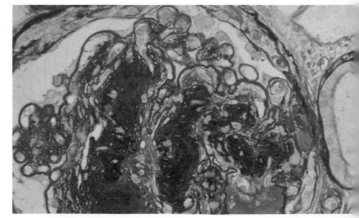

Fig. 17. Haematoxylin and eosin stain of renal glomerulus from a diabetic patient with persistent proteinuria. Loss of normal histological architecture and basement membrane thickening can be seen.

Assessing the newly diagnosed patient for cardiovascular disease
• Careful history, eg exertional chest pain, cigarette smoking and alcohol intake
• Physical examination: evidence of end-organ damage, eg left ventricular hypertrophy, retinal changes, absent peripheral pulses, neck and femoral bruits
• Risk factor screening: Blood pressure measurement - every visit Lipid profile - total and HDL cholesterol (fasting triglycerides) HbA$_{1c}$ Serum creatinine Proteinuria Timed overnight urine collection (albumin excretion rate) or albumin/creatinine ratio on a spot specimen of urine 12-lead ECG Coronary heart disease risk assessment
• Where indicated: exercise ECG, echocardiogram and chest x-ray

and hypertrophy. Co-existing hypertension will exacerbate these problems.

Heart failure is a result of left ventricular diastolic dysfunction or combined left ventricular diastolic and systolic dysfunction. This type of problem has been described as "dilated cardiomyopathy" and is associated with increased risk of sudden death, perhaps related to ventricular arrhythmia. These problems are compounded in the diabetic patient by microvascular involvement of the myocardium, infiltration of the conducting system and right ventricular dysfunction.

Fig. 18. Initial assessment of the newly diagnosed patient with type 2 diabetes for vascular diasease.

Diagnosis

As diabetes is a cardiovascular disease, screening and aggressive intervention for all cardiovascular risk factors is essential. At presentation around 50% of type 2 diabetic patients show evidence of cardiovascular disease, so part of initial assessment must include the points outlined in Figure 18.

Coronary heart disease risk should also be assessed. This takes into account the influence of major coronary heart disease risk factors for an individual and their annual expression in terms of 5- or 10-year risk. The widest used tool is the equation based on the Framingham study, which can be calculated on computer

66 Screening and aggressive intervention for all cardiovascular risk factors is essential in diabetes 99

" Of some dispute is the level of coronary heart disease risk at which intervention is required "

programmes.[31] The equation takes into account the factors shown in Figure 19.

The calculation is valid for people aged 30 to 74 years only and is used as a tool for primary prevention. It does not apply to those with ischaemic heart disease or genetic dyslipidaemias.

In addition, the data entry only includes classical factors and does not take into account other important issues such as ethnic origin (for example, Asians are at higher risk), presence of proteinuria or family history of heart disease.

Of some dispute is the level of coronary heart disease risk at which intervention is required. For example, the initial advice of the Government's Standing Medical Advisory Committee in the UK suggested drug treatment for individuals in whom the 10-year risk was greater than 30%.[32] This equates to an overall cardiovascular risk (including stroke) of around 40%, which many feel is much too high. More recent guidelines from the Joint British Societies, British Hypertension Society, WHO and the National Institute for Clinical Excellence have lowered the threshold to greater than 15% risk of coronary heart disease over 10 years.[33]

Prevention of cardiovascular disease

Until recently, hard evidence for risk factor intervention to reduce risk of cardiovascular morbidity and mortality was unavailable for patients with diabetes. Previously, this evidence had to be extrapolated from large trials conducted in the general population, some of

Fig. 19. Risk factors commonly used to calculate coronary heart disease risk in appropriate patients aged 30 to 74 years.[31]

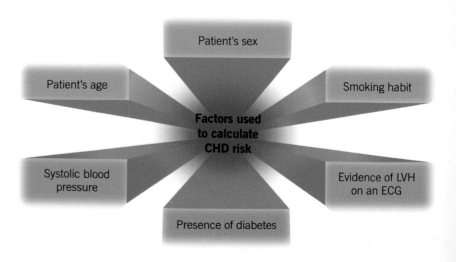

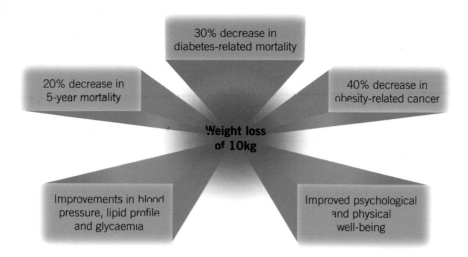

which included patients with diabetes. The situation has now changed dramatically.

Fig. 20. Impact of 10kg weight loss in an obese patient.

Evidence base for treatment
Obesity

The effect of weight loss of 10kg in an obese patient is shown in Figure 20.[34] Weight loss in diabetic patients may be difficult, partly because of the nature of the disease itself, but also because some of the treatments for glycaemia may promote weight gain, for example sulphonylureas and insulin. Despite this, even modest weight loss of 5% to 10% may be associated with significant benefit. Several studies have supported the benefits of weight loss in preventing/delaying the onset of type 2 diabetes in patients with impaired glucose tolerance.[35,36]

These studies demonstrated that the single most important factor in diabetes prevention is weight loss, with 50% to 60% reductions in conversion from impaired glucose tolerance to type 2 diabetes (Figure 21).

Potentially even more interesting are the results from the recent XENDOS (Xenical (orlistat) and prevention of Diabetes in Obese Subjects) trial, which at the time of writing are yet to be published. This four-year Swedish multicentre study involved over 3000 participants. The patients were obese with a BMI over 30kg/m² and only a fifth had impaired glucose tolerance at the time of entry. All patients received advice on a mildly hypocaloric diet and moderate physical activity. In addition, they were randomized to receive either orlistat 120mg, three times a day, or placebo.

" Weight loss in diabetic patients may be difficult because some treatments for glycaemia may promote weight gain "

21

Trial	Intervention	Mean follow up (years)	↓ Progression
Da Qing[154] (577 patients)	Diet alone v control	6.0	31%
	Exercise alone v control	6.0	46%
	Diet + exercise v control	6.0	42%
DPS[35] (522 patients)	Diet + exercise v control	3.2	58%
DPP[36] (3234 patients)	Diet + exercise v standard	2.8	58%

Fig. 21. Lifestyle intervention reduces risk of progression of impaired glucose tolerance to type 2 diabetes.

"Risk of diabetes development was reduced by 37% in patients treated with orlistat"

The risk of diabetes development was reduced by 37% in those treated with orlistat compared with those given lifestyle modification alone. This is likely to be accounted for by the fact that weight loss was greater in those who received orlistat than in those on lifestyle modification alone (-6.9kg versus -4.1kg over 4 years). This reduction was also associated with significant falls in LDL cholesterol (-12.8% versus -5.1%) and blood pressure (-4.9mmHg versus -3.4mmHg) in those treated with orlistat compared with placebo.

In those with established type 2 diabetes a retrospective study demonstrated an average weight loss of 1kg was associated with increased survival of 3 to 4 months.[37] Extrapolation suggests a 10kg weight loss would restore around a third of the life expectancy in obese type 2 diabetic patients to reach the figure in the healthy population.

As well as improving the classical cardiovascular risk factors in type 2 diabetes, weight loss is also associated with improvements in:[28]

"A 10kg weight loss would restore around a third of the life expectancy in an obese type 2 diabetic patient"

- intravascular blood volume
- cardiac pressures
- sympathetic activity
- insulin resistance.

Glycaemia

The United Kingdom Prospective Diabetes Study (UKPDS) randomized over 5000 patients newly diagnosed with type 2 diabetes to a regime of either tight or conventional diabetic control.[38] During the 20-year study period the investigators achieved a separation of glycate haemoglobin (HbA$_{1c}$) of 7.0% versus 7.9% in favour of tight control. This was associated with significant relative risk reductions for microvascular and any diabetes-related end points and a non-significant risk reduction for myocardial infarction (Figure 22). Epidemiological extrapolation suggests that for every 1% reduction in HbA$_{1c}$ profound benefit, including reduction in cardiovascular events, would be expected.

> *For every 1% reduction in HbA$_{1c}$, profound benefit would be expected*

This major and important prospective study supports a range of earlier retrospective studies that have shown a strong relationship between glycaemia and risk of vascular disease.

Hypertension

The UKPDS had a large sub-group of hypertensive patients. These too were randomized into a tight and conventional blood pressure treatment group, and over 9 years a separation in systolic pressure of 10mmHg and diastolic pressure of 5mmHg was achieved in favour of tight blood pressure control.[39] This was associated with profound vascular benefit with significant reductions in microvascular end points, diabetes-related end points, death related to diabetes and stroke more dramatic even than that shown for tight glycaemic control (Figure 22).

Fig. 22. Summary of glycaemia and blood pressure data from the UK Prospective Diabetes Study.[38,39]

Glycaemia: Tight (HbA$_{1c}$ 7%) versus conventional (HbA$_{1c}$ 7.9%) control		
	↓RR (%)	*p* value
Microvascular end point	25	0.010
Myocardial infarction	16	0.052
Any diabetes-related end point	12	0.029

Blood pressure: Tight (mean 144/82mmHg) versus conventional (mean 154/87mmHg) control		
	↓RR (%)	*p* value
Microvascular end points	37	0.010
Diabetes-related end points	24	0.005
Deaths related to diabetes	32	0.020
Stroke	44	0.013
↓RR = relative risk reduction		

66 *To achieve target blood pressure, two or more antihypertensive agents from different classes are normally required* 99

This data is supported by results from the Hypertension Optimal Treatment (HOT) study.[40] Around 19,000 patients aged 50 to 80 years with a diastolic blood pressure of 100mmHg to 115mmHg were randomized to target diastolic blood pressures of less than 80, 85 or 90mmHg. A significant 51% reduction in major cardiovascular events in the group with a target blood pressure of less than 80mmHg compared with the less than 90mmHg group was seen in the subset of 1500 patients with diabetes (Figure 23). The HOT study also demonstrated the benefits of low-dose aspirin with a significant reduction in cardiovascular end points and mortality in those treated with this therapy (although at the expense of an increased risk of non-fatal haemorrhagic episodes).

Both the UKPDS and HOT studies clearly demonstrated that to achieve target blood pressure, two or more antihypertensive agents

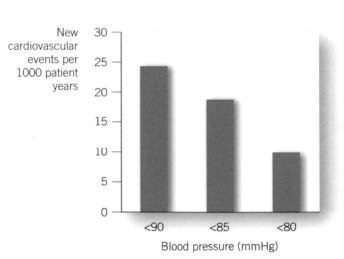

Fig. 23. The HOT study demonstrated halving of cardiovascular end points and mortality in the group randomized to "tight" compared with "least tight" blood pressure control.

from different classes were normally required. In the HOT study, around two-thirds of patients in the most intensively treated group required two or more agents.

Six large randomized prospective trials have now confirmed the considerable benefit of antihypertensive treatment on cardiovascular outcomes in diabetic patients, including the two already mentioned. In the Systolic Hypertension in the Elderly Programme (SHEP)[41] around 600 elderly patients with diabetes were included. The study was placebo controlled and patients were allocated to receive treatment with a thiazide diuretic, with or without atenolol or reserpine. There was around a 10mmHg reduction in systolic pressure compared with the control group with a reduction in relative risk of myocardial infarction of 46%.

In the Systolic Hypertension in Europe (SYST-EUR) trial a sub-group analysis of almost 500 diabetic patients with hypertension demonstrated that calcium channel blocker based therapy was associated with reductions of 55% in total mortality, 76% in cardiovascular mortality and 73% in stroke compared with placebo.[42]

Benefits of using antihypertensives that specifically block the renin-angiotensin system have recently been demonstrated by the Captopril Prevention Project (CAPPP)[43] and the Heart Outcomes Prevention Evaluation (HOPE) study[44] in diabetic patients. Significant reductions in cardiovascular event rates and mortality were shown compared with standard treatments.

The evidence demonstrates unequivocally that good blood pressure control in diabetic patients is vital as it will dramatically reduce the risk of cardiovascular morbidity and total mortality.

❝ Good blood pressure control in diabetic patients is vital as it will dramatically reduce the risk of cardiovascular morbidity and total mortality ❞

Dyslipidaemia

Six trials have unequivocally demonstrated the profound benefits of statin therapy in reducing cardiovascular morbidity and mortality, from the point of view of both primary and secondary prevention.[45-50]

The first five trials demonstrated that lowering serum cholesterol by around 20% reduced the relative risk of coronary heart disease by approximately one third. The benefits have been shown for both secondary and primary prevention for both sexes up to age 75. Unfortunately, relatively few diabetic patients were involved, and in only one trial was there enough power for a subgroup analysis to be performed and demonstrate statistically significant benefit.[51] The diabetic cohort in the 4S programme[45] did at least as well as the non-diabetic patients with statin treatment.

Recently, the Heart Protection Study, which included almost 4000 patients with diabetes, without clinically evident cardiovascular disease, has provided direct evidence for a major role for such therapy in the primary prevention of cardiovascular disease in diabetic patients.[50]

The Heart Protection Study included over 20,000 patients, one fifth being diabetic, and was set up to determine the effect of lowering cholesterol with a statin (simvastatin) in patients at higher risk of cardiovascular disease. Patients had to have pre-existing cardiovascular disease or be at high risk because of diabetes or hypertension. The lower limit of entry for the trial was a serum cholesterol of 3.5mmol/l.

❝ Six trials have unequivocally demonstrated the profound benefits of statin therapy in reducing cardiovascular morbidity and mortality ❞

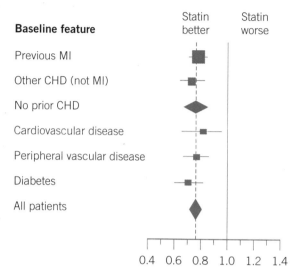

Risk ratio and 95% confidence interval

Baseline feature	Statin better	Statin worse
Previous MI		
Other CHD (not MI)		
No prior CHD		
Cardiovascular disease		
Peripheral vascular disease		
Diabetes		
All patients		

0.4 0.6 0.8 1.0 1.2 1.4

66 Statins could and should be given to all patients at high cardiovascular risk 99

Fig. 24. Vascular event by prior disease with simvastatin in the Heart Protection Study. In diabetic patients event rates were reduced by around one third. All numbers to the left of the vertical line indicate a significant reduction in events in the statin treatment group. For example, the figure for the diabetic patients is around 0.7 on this scale, indicating a 30% relative risk reduction from unity. Reproduced from Heart Protection Study Collaborative Group. Lancet 2002;360: 7-22 with permission from Elsevier.

All patients in the active group received a fixed daily dose of 40mg of simvastatin, with no titration against serum cholesterol concentration.

Over the 5 years of the study statin therapy was associated with:

- relative risk reduction for coronary heart disease of approximately one third in both diabetic and non-diabetic patients (Figure 24)
- the same relative risk reduction at all levels of serum cholesterol (Figure 25)
- benefit up to 80 years of age
- reduced risk not just for coronary heart disease but also for peripheral vascular disease, stroke and transient ischaemic attacks.

What the Heart Protection Study also tells us is that the approach to cholesterol lowering to a target of total serum cholesterol of less than 5mmol/l and/or LDL to less than 3mmol/l is incorrect. Opinion

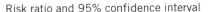

Risk ratio and 95% confidence interval

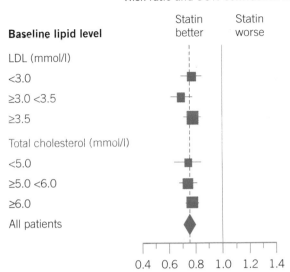

Fig. 25. Vascular event by prior lipid levels with simvastatin in the Heart Protection Study. Shows the same degree of benefit at all levels of cholesterol. All numbers to the left of the vertical line indicate a significant reduction in events in the statin treatment group. For example, the figure for the diabetic patients is around 0.7 on this scale, indicating a 30% relative risk reduction from unity. Reproduced from Heart Protection Study Collaborative Group. Lancet 2002;360: 7-22 with permission from Elsevier.

is now increasingly that statins could and should be given to all patients at high cardiovascular risk whatever their level of serum cholesterol, including diabetic patients.

This has recently been recognized by the National Institute for Clinical Excellence guidance on treatment of dyslipidaemia in diabetes, which now recommends intervention with a statin at a 15% 10-year coronary heart disease risk at any level of cholesterol – in other words the significant majority of patients with type 2 diabetes.[33] This will have major pharmacoeconomic implications.

66 NICE guidance on treatment of dyslipidaemia in diabetes will have major pharmacoeconomic implications 99

Summary
There is now an excellent evidence base for managing the major cardiovascular risk factors in diabetic patients with evidence-based targets as outlined in Figure 26.[52,53]

Evidence-based targets for managing cardiovascular risk factors

• Fasting blood glucose	≤ 6mmol/l
• HbA$_{1c}$	< 7%
• Total cholesterol	< 5mmol/l
• LDL cholesterol	< 3mmol/l
• Blood pressure threshold for intervention	140/90mmHg
- target for treatment	≤ 140/80mmHg
- if significant proteinuria	≤ 125/75mmHg

- Recent guidelines recommend statin and low-dose aspirin treatment where the 10-year coronary heart disease risk is less than 15%
  - before adding aspirin ensure blood pressure is controlled
  - combination antihypertensive treatment is necessary in the majority of patients to achieve blood pressure targets
  - other recommendations include HDL >1.2mmol/l and fasting triglycerides <1.7mmol/l

Fig. 26. Summary of treatment targets for cardiovascular risk factor intervention in diabetic patients.

Treatment

This book will focus on managing cardiovascular risk factors emphasizing, in particular, the multiprofessional and multiple risk factor intervention approach to reducing cardiovascular morbidity and mortality.

The holistic approach to diabetes management must include:
- advice on the importance of weight loss
- dietary changes
- increased physical activity
- cessation of cigarette smoking and
- reduction of alcohol intake where indicated.

Obesity

Any weight management programme must include advice on increased physical activity and reduction in caloric intake. Weight reduction can be associated with profound health benefits. The objectives of obesity management are shown in Figure 27.

Weight management programmes can be successful in the short term and may be helped by anti-obesity drugs. In the past, these agents have had a bad press because of side-effects, but recently a new type of anti-obesity agent, orlistat, has become available.[54]

66 Any weight management programme must include advice on increased physical activity and reduction in caloric intake 99

This works by competitive inhibition of pancreatic and intestinal lipase preventing the breakdown of about 30% of ingested fat.

Orlistat should be used where the patient has demonstrated a commitment to weight loss, including the ability to lose 2.5kg in the month before drug treatment.

The licence suggests continuing drug treatment beyond 3 months only if more than 5% of total body weight is lost, although in diabetic patients one can afford to be more flexible because of profound benefits resulting from any degree of weight loss. The drug should be given as part of a weight management programme, and providing dietary recommendations are followed side-effects, such as oily stool, are not usually a problem.

Two-year studies have demonstrated significant weight loss and much less weight gain compared with placebo, and this is associated with a significant reduction in abdominal circumference and improvements in glycaemia and other cardiovascular risk factors.[54]

Although weight loss is not as profound in diabetic patients, improvement in blood pressure and metabolic parameters may be particularly marked.

Another agent, sibutramine, has also recently been licensed.[55] This centrally acting drug is also associated with significant weight loss as part of a weight management programme, and has shown similar benefits to those described above.

There are, however, concerns about development of hypertension in some patients so these agents need to be used with caution in diabetes.

" In diabetic patients one can afford to be more flexible because of the profound benefits resulting from any degree of weight loss "

Fig. 27. Objectives of obesity management.

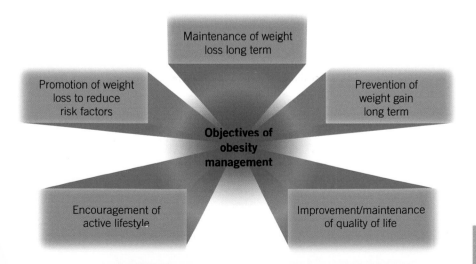

Glycaemia

The benefits of improved glycaemic control were well demonstrated by the UK Prospective Diabetes Study, which showed marked risk reductions for diabetic microvascular disease and other diabetes-related end points.[38] Unfortunately, this study did not show significant reduction in risk for cardiovascular events, although reduction in myocardial infarction rate almost reached significance. Epidemiological extrapolation, however, suggests that such benefits would have been achieved with better separation of HbA_{1c} between the two groups.

There are several classes of anti-diabetic agents that can be used to improve glycaemia (Figure 28).

Fig. 28. Anti-diabetic agents that can be used to improve glycaemia.

Drug classes used to improve glycaemia	
• Biguanides	• Thiazolidinediones (glitazones)
• Sulphonylureas	• Rapid-acting secretagogues
• Alpha-glucosidase inhibitors	• Insulins

Biguanides

The only example in use is metformin, which reduces hepatic glucose output and has a mild insulin-sensitizing effect. It is wise to start with a low dose, with gradual build up over several months to maintenance levels, taking the drug on a full stomach as otherwise incidence of gastrointestinal side-effects may be high. The drug is efficacious in improving glycaemia and has been shown to be associated with a reduction in risk of cardiovascular morbidity and mortality.[56] For this reason it should normally be the first-line oral antidiabetic agent in all diabetic patients with a BMI of $25kg/m^2$ or higher.

> ❝ *Metformin should normally be the first-line oral antidiabetic agent* ❞

Sulphonylureas

These include glibenclamide, gliclazide, glipizide and glimepiride, and promote insulin secretion from the beta cells of the pancreas.[57] They are efficacious in improving glycaemia but may be associated with weight gain and hypoglycaemia. The latter is particularly the case for the longer-acting drugs, such as glibenclamide, which should be avoided in the elderly. These agents are recommended as second line in combination with metformin in patients with an HbA_{1c} over 7%.

Alpha-glucosidase inhibitors

The only agent on the market in the UK is acarbose, which competitively inhibits breakdown of long-chain sugars to glucose in the gut.[58] It works principally by reducing postprandial hyperglycaemia and has only limited efficacy in reducing HbA_{1c}. It is normally used in combination with other oral agents but many patients discontinue because of gastrointestinal side-effects.

Thiazolidinediones (glitazones)

Given that insulin resistance is a fundamental defect of type 2 diabetes (Figure 29) and associated with increased cardiovascular risk, the advent of the thiazolidinediones (glitazones) has caused much interest. This is because these agents improve insulin sensitivity, thereby reducing insulin resistance.

The need for new oral agents for type 2 diabetes

The most widely used oral agents for managing type 2 diabetes include metformin (normally first line) or sulphonylureas, or a combination of the two. These drugs have been around for many years and were used in the United Kingdom Prospective Diabetes Study,[38] which demonstrated the value of tight glycaemic control in reducing vascular (principally microvascular) risk. Unfortunately, none of the traditional oral agents, including insulin, appears to affect disease progression, and even in the tightly controlled group there was a gradual deterioration in glycaemic control over time.

In addition, metformin can cause gastrointestinal side-effects and sulphonylureas and insulin are associated with weight gain and risk of hypoglycaemia. Also, none of the traditional oral agents directly targets the primary defects of type 2 diabetes, although metformin does have a mild insulin-sensitizing effect.

> **None of the traditional oral agents directly targets the primary defects of type 2 diabetes**

> **The advent of the thiazolidinediones has caused much interest**

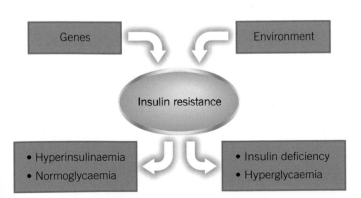

Fig. 29. A combination of insulin resistance and pancreatic β-cell secretory defect are normally required for development of type 2 diabetes.

For all these reasons there has been much interest in approaches to diabetes management that more directly target the primary defects of the condition. The long-term hope is that this will not only improve blood glucose control but will also slow or prevent progression of the disease and reduce cardiovascular risk.

Mechanism of action of glitazones

These agents combine with an intranuclear hormone receptor called peroxisome proliferator activated receptor gamma (PPARγ).[59] This combination produces effects on carbohydrate and lipid metabolism, fat cell differentiation and gene regulation similar to that seen when insulin combines with its receptor (Figure 30). These agents are therefore insulin sparing, improving insulin sensitivity and thereby reducing insulin resistance.

Animal data with these agents was extremely interesting, demonstrating significant improvements to glucose and the lipid profile, improving insulin resistance, attenuation or prevention of diabetic nephropathy and prevention of pancreatic islet cell degeneration.[60]

Fig. 30. Mode of action of thiazolidinedione drugs, which "sensitise" the body to naturally produced insulin.

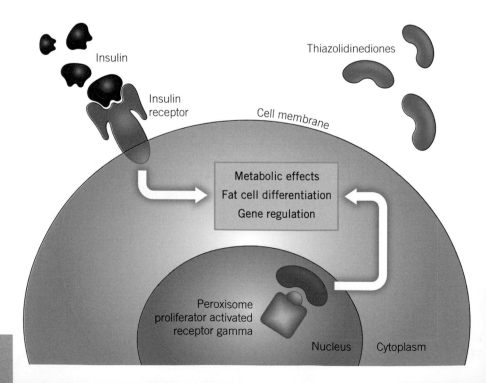

Insulin

Thiazolidinediones

Insulin receptor

Cell membrane

Metabolic effects
Fat cell differentiation
Gene regulation

Peroxisome proliferator activated receptor gamma

Nucleus   Cytoplasm

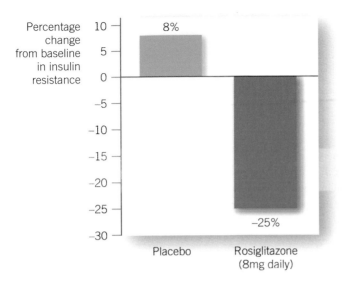

Percentage change from baseline in insulin resistance

Placebo — 8%

Rosiglitazone (8mg daily) — −25%

Fig. 31. Improvement in insulin resistance (based on HOMA analysis) over 6 months in patients with type 2 diabetes with rosiglitazone compared with placebo. Reproduced from Matthews DR et al. Rosiglitazone decreases insulin resistance and improves beta-cell function in patients with type 2 diabetes. Diabetologia 1999;42(Suppl 1):A228 with permission from Springer-Verlag.

Clinical trial data

The first glitazone to come to market (troglitazone) was eventually withdrawn because of idiosyncratic hepatotoxic reactions, which in some cases led to liver failure and death in around one in 60,000 patients.[59] The more recently introduced agents, rosiglitazone (Avandia, GlaxoSmithKline) and pioglitazone (Actos, Takeda UK Ltd), do not have these problems. Both have been on the market in the US for some years, and more recently in Europe.

Clinical trials have clearly demonstrated improvements in insulin sensitivity (Figure 31). This has been demonstrated in placebo-controlled comparisons and in glitazone combination studies with either metformin or sulphonylureas.[61]

The homeostasis model assessment (HOMA) method of analysis has been used. This is a simple and validated model for measuring both insulin sensitivity/resistance and beta cell function. Improvement in beta cell function is also supported by the fact that insulin, proinsulin and split proinsulin products are all reduced compared with placebo or other oral agents in studies of up to 52 weeks.[62]

The fact there is an improvement in glycaemia at the same time as a reduction in circulating insulin levels also supports the contention that there is an improvement in insulin sensitivity with these agents.

Both pioglitazone and rosiglitazone monotherapy studies versus placebo have demonstrated falls in fasting plasma glucose of 2mmol/l to 3mmol/l and a reduction of HbA$_{1c}$ of around 1% compared with

66 Pioglitazone and rosiglitazone monotherapy studies versus placebo have demonstrated falls in fasting plasma glucose of 2–3mmol/l 99

Fig. 32. The glitazone, pioglitazone, in combination with either sulphonylurea or metformin is associated with around 1% improvement in HbA$_{1c}$ over 4 months. Reproduced from Einhorn D. Pioglitazone hydrochloride in combination with metformin in the treatment of type 2 diabetes mellitus: a randomized, placebo-controlled study. Clinical Therapeutics 2000;22:1395 with permission from Elsevier.

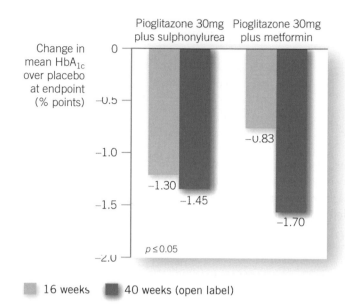

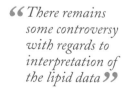

placebo (Figure 32).[59] Glitazones take 2 to 3 months to achieve maximal effect and the eventual magnitude of the fall is similar to that seen with traditional agents. Indeed, the longer-term studies have reported sustained control of up to 30 months.[63]

Combination studies with either metformin or sulphonylurea lasting between 16 and 26 weeks demonstrated a further improvement of around 1% in HbA$_{1c}$ when adding a glitazone compared with these agents alone.[59] Several studies have also looked at insulin/glitazone combinations in patients with type 2 diabetes.[64] These people tend to be very insulin resistant and so this is a logical approach. Trial data has demonstrated improvement in HbA$_{1c}$ and also the possibility of significant reduction in insulin dose.

> *66 There remains some controversy with regards to interpretation of the lipid data 99*

Glitazones and other parameters of the metabolic syndrome
The glitazones produce a significant reduction in circulating free fatty acids regulated partly by stimulation of lipogenesis via PPARγ. Beyond this, there remains some controversy about interpretation of the lipid data. Type 2 diabetic patients typically have low HDL cholesterol and raised triglycerides. Troglitazone and pioglitazone reduced triglycerides significantly in clinical trials but this was less marked with rosiglitazone.[59,65] The patient groups studied may not, however, have been strictly comparable and subgroup analysis of the rosiglitazone data suggests patients with higher levels of triglycerides may show a reduction.

There also appears to be an initial increase in LDL cholesterol, followed by a later increase in HDL cholesterol in several clinical trials. Overall, an improvement in the total cholesterol to HDL cholesterol ratio (which should benefit arterial disease) has been demonstrated.

The idea that glitazone use is associated with an improvement in the lipid profile is supported by studies looking at lipoprotein density where there is a shift from the small, dense, atherogenic lipoproteins to the light, fluffy, less atherogenic particles.[66]

These agents also appear to be associated with a small, but significant reduction in blood pressure. In one 52-week study, using ambulatory blood pressure monitoring[67] comparing glibenclamide with rosiglitazone, there was a significant increase in systolic pressure in the sulphonylurea group, but no change in the rosiglitazone group (Figure 33). For diastolic blood pressure there was no change in the sulphonylurea group but a significant 2mmHg reduction in the rosiglitazone group.

From the point of view of other parameters associated with the metabolic syndrome, there are preliminary reports of a beneficial effect of glitazones on albumin excretion rate compared with sulphonylureas

66 There are reports of a beneficial effect of glitazones on albumin excretion rate 99

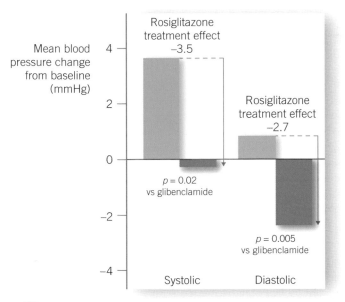

Fig. 33. The glitazones have been associated with improvements in blood pressure when compared with standard therapy in patients with type 2 diabetes over 52 weeks. This may relate to their insulin sensitizing effect. Reproduced from Diabetes Care 2002;25:2058-64 with permission from the American Diabetes Association.

Glibenclamide (mean dose 10.5mg/day) (n=66)

Rosiglitazone monotherapy 4mg BD (n=63)

in microalbuminuric type 2 diabetic patients, reduction in inflammatory markers such as C-reactive protein and down regulation of plasminogen activator inhibitor-1, all suggesting an improvement in the atherogenic risk profile.[59]

66 Generally glitazones appear to have a good side-effect profile 99

Safety

The concern that rosiglitazone and pioglitazone might cause similar idiosyncratic hepatotoxic reactions to those shown with troglitazone has not been borne out. The extensive clinical trial programme and the fact that glitazones have been used in well over 5 million people in the US without any sign of liver problems is testimony to this.

Generally glitazones appear to have a good side-effect profile and do not increase risks of hypoglycaemia or cause gastrointestinal side-effects. They may, however, be associated with weight gain of around 3kg to 4kg in the first 6 months of treatment which then tends to stabilize.[59] This is in part due to redistribution of fat from central stores (intrahepatic and visceral fat) to peripheral fat stores, which in the context of metabolic syndrome may actually be a good thing. Certainly, any weight gain is not associated with significant deterioration in cardiovascular risk parameters.

The main safety issues relate to fluid retention. The exact mechanism of this is unknown, but around 5% of patients will show some evidence of peripheral oedema.[59] This rarely necessitates drug withdrawal, may be self-limiting and is easily treated. There is, however, a theoretical possibility of precipitating heart failure or worsening the condition in predisposed individuals. For these reasons, glitazones are contraindicated in Europe in patients with a current or past history of heart failure, although the restrictions in the US are less rigorous with contraindications only in the more severe cases.

66 Studies are also underway to determine whether glitazones may be valuable in preventing development of type 2 diabetes in those with impaired glucose tolerance 99

A few patients will develop anaemia based on a fall of about 1g haemoglobin. This is a class effect occurring within the first 6 months of treatment. This is due to haemodilution and is not a true anaemia. There is no evidence of bone marrow suppression or any effects on red cell turnover or the oxygen carrying capacity of the blood.[68]

Licence restrictions in Europe

Licensing conditions are much more restrictive in Europe than in the US. In Europe they can only be used in combination with sulphonylureas or metformin. In other words, in obese patients in combination with metformin with insufficient glycaemic control, or in sulphonylurea-treated patients where metformin is contraindicated or not tolerated. They are also contraindicated in combination with insulin and in patients with a history of heart failure. In the US they can be used not

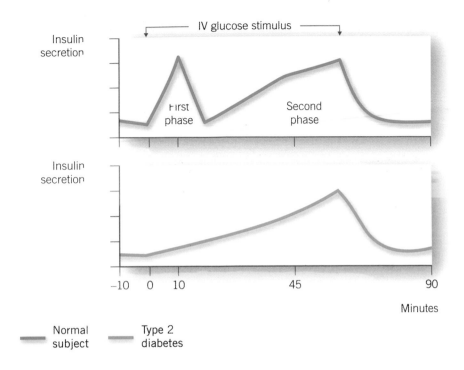

Normal subject — Type 2 diabetes

only in combination with other oral agents but also as monotherapy and in combination with insulin. Clinical trials are ongoing to support a change of licence in Europe with far fewer restrictions.

The future

Long-term clinical trials are underway that look at hard end points, including those relating to cardiovascular disease and mortality, to see whether the theoretical possibility that glitazones might reduce cardiovascular risk by improving insulin resistance is indeed the case. The trials will also determine whether glitazones affect disease progression by providing sustained control in the long term. Studies are also underway to determine whether these agents may be valuable in preventing development of type 2 diabetes in those with impaired glucose tolerance. If these trials are positive then the glitazones would have decided advantages over traditional agents.

Several new drugs are also being studied that are agonists of both PPARγ and PPARα. In theory, these agents should have similar beneficial effects to those seen with the glitazones, which act on PPARγ. In addition, stimulation of PPARα is predicted to cause more profound reduction in triglycerides and increased HDL in a similar fashion to that seen with the fibrate group of drugs, which are predominantly agonists of PPARα.

Fig. 34. Insulin response to intravenous glucose in a person with normal glucose tolerance and in a person with type 2 diabetes. The latter has total loss of first (early) phase insulin secretion.

Rapid-acting insulin secretagogues

Although insulin resistance is a fundamental feature in the development of type 2 diabetes, it is not the only pathophysiological defect. Indeed, both insulin resistance and beta cell deficiency are normally required for type 2 diabetes to develop.

One of the earliest features of type 2 diabetes, and indeed seen in the pre-diabetic phase, is loss of early-phase insulin secretion (Figure 34, p37).[69] Early-phase insulin secretion is seen after a meal or after oral or intravenous ingestion of glucose. It is responsible for inhibition of hepatic glucose output and its absence results in postprandial hyperglycaemia. Traditional oral hypoglycaemic agents tend to target fasting hyperglycaemia, but it has become apparent that both fasting and postprandial hyperglycaemia contribute to overall glycaemic burden and therefore to total HbA_{1c}.[70] Progressive failure of pancreatic beta cells occurs whether patients are obese or non-obese and appears not to be affected by traditional agents for the management of type 2 diabetes.

> *It has become apparent that both fasting and postprandial hyperglycaemia contribute to overall glycaemic burden and therefore to total HbA_{1c}*

Postprandial hyperglycaemia and cardiovascular risk

As already discussed, cardiovascular disease is by far the commonest cause of morbidity and mortality in patients with type 2 diabetes. Although this excess mortality occurs in part because of co-occurrence of other cardiovascular risk factors, diabetes is itself an independent and important primary risk factor.

There is a large body of evidence that relates postprandial hyperglycaemia to cardiovascular outcomes and mortality.[69] Although several studies have shown this association, it was not until the Diabetes Epidemiology: Collaborative Analysis of Diagnostic Criteria in Europe (DECODE) study was published in 1999 that people really started to take notice.[71] The DECODE study looked at the relationship between fasting and postprandial hyperglycaemia on total mortality and morbidity. Data in over 25,000 patients demonstrated that post-challenge glucose was better and more sensitive than fasting glucose in predicting risk of mortality (Figure 35).

Whether this association is causal is still hotly debated. For example, postprandial hyperglycaemia is also associated with postprandial hyperlipidaemia, which has been associated with increased oxidative stress and endothelial dysfunction. Both have been implicated in the atherogenic process.[72,73]

What is clear, is that much more work needs to be done in this area. One could postulate, however, that agents which more directly target postprandial hyperglycaemia might not only play a role in managing type 2 diabetes, but offer the tantalizing possibility of reducing cardiovascular risk.

Two rapid-acting insulin secretagogues that target postprandial hyperglycaemia have recently come on the market: repaglinide (NovoNorm, Novonordisk) and nateglinide (Starlix, Novartis).

Repaglinide

Repaglinide is structurally related to meglitinide and is actually derived from the non-sulphonylurea portion of glibenclamide.[69] It binds to the sulphonylurea receptor and to its own distinct binding site on the beta

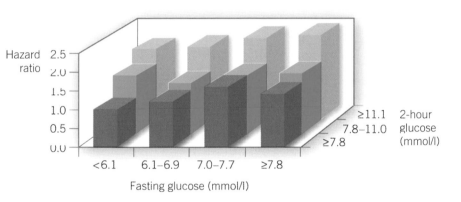

Fasting glucose (mmol/l)

cell. It acts in a similar fashion to sulphonylureas (provoking closure of ATP-sensitive potassium channels) but has a very rapid onset and short duration of action. For this reason, it is taken immediately before a meal. Clinical trials have demonstrated a 2% reduction in HbA_{1c}, a fall in fasting glucose of around 4mmol/l and in postprandial glucose of around 6mmol/l in treatment-naive patients compared with placebo.[71]

Repaglinide has also been used in combination with metformin, and compared with metformin treatment alone is associated with falls of HbA_{1c} in excess of 1% and fasting glucose of 2mmol/l.[75]

Because of its rapid action and short duration of effect this agent may be associated with a reduced risk of hypoglycaemia and less weight gain than with traditional sulphonylureas.[76,77]

Use of repaglinide in combination with insulin has also been reported.[69] One study demonstrated that the combination of repaglinide with bedtime isophane insulin resulted in additional reduction in HbA_{1c} of around 1.7% compared with bedtime isophane alone.[78] This is similar data to that seen with a sulphonylurea/insulin combination, but the prolonged hyperinsulinaemia and increased risk of hypoglycaemia may be a disadvantage of the latter when used in this way.

Fig. 35. Mean plus 95% confidence intervals for death according to fasting glucose and 2-hour glucose in individuals not known to have diabetes. The hazard ratio for death is significantly greater based on 2-hour postprandial glucose values compared with fasting glucose. Reproduced from Lancet 1999;354:617-21 with permission from Elsevier.

39

Nateglinide

Nateglinide has no sulphonylurea moiety and is derived from an amino acid – phenylalanine (Figure 36).[69] Although it acts similarly to repaglinide and sulphonylureas by inhibiting pancreatic beta-cell potassium ATP-sensitive channels, there are also significant differences. These include the fact that nateglinide's residency time on the receptor is a few seconds, rather than the several minutes seen with repaglinide and sulphonylureas. This is probably why it has a faster onset and shorter duration of action than the other insulin secretagogues, including repaglinide.

The result is a very rapid onset and short duration rise in insulin levels which peak soon after taking the drug. Nateglinide is also glucose sensitive in that the drug does not elicit a significant rise in insulin levels unless a meal is eaten.[79]

The principle action of nateglinide is to reduce postprandial hyperglycaemia with significantly less effect on fasting glucose compared with sulphonylureas.[69] The postprandial rise in insulin levels after

> **❝** *Nateglinide is particularly useful where there are concerns about hypoglycaemia and weight gain* **❞**

Fig. 36. The structure of nateglinide, a rapid-acting insulin secretagogue derived from an amino acid (phenylalanine).

D-phenylalanine

nateglinide is more physiological with a fine peak and rapid loss of insulin from the circulation resulting in less hyperinsulinaemia between meals. This results in significantly reduced risk of hypoglycaemia and weight gain compared with sulphonylureas.[80,81]

The best way to use this agent is in combination with metformin, because metformin more directly targets fasting glucose (Figure 37). The combination results in more profound reductions in HbA_{1c} than seen with either agent alone. The combination was also associated with a very low risk of hypoglycaemia and hardly any weight gain over a 6-month period.

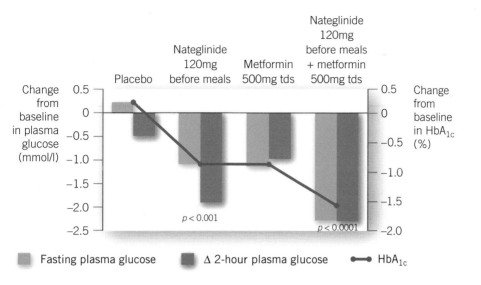

| | Placebo | Nateglinide 120mg before meals | Metformin 500mg tds | Nateglinide 120mg before meals + metformin 500mg tds |

Change from baseline in plasma glucose (mmol/l)

Change from baseline in HbA₁c (%)

$p < 0.001$

$p < 0.0001$

■ Fasting plasma glucose ■ Δ 2-hour plasma glucose ●— HbA₁c

Nateglinide is therefore useful in type 2 diabetic patients, particularly where there are concerns about hypoglycaemia and weight gain, and appears safer in "missed meal" situations where the insulin response is much attenuated after the drug compared with sulphonylureas.

This type of agent may also be particularly useful in the early phases of the disease (although it is only licensed for metformin combination) and even in the phase of impaired glucose tolerance. There is also the tantalizing possibility that by reducing postprandial hyperglycaemia there could be a reduction in risk of cardiovascular disease, although this needs further study and remains a hypothesis. Ongoing studies both from the point of view of cardiovascular disease and in patients with impaired glucose tolerance should answer these questions in the next few years.

Insulin therapy

Although the value of tight diabetic control in reducing long-term risk of microvascular complications has been unequivocally demonstrated by the Diabetes Control and Complications Trial[82] in type 1 diabetes and the UK Prospective Diabetes Study[38] in type 2 diabetes, such control is difficult to achieve in many patients and there may be a price to pay from the point of view of increased risk of hypoglycaemia.

Injectable insulin preparations rarely achieve adequate glycaemic control because they do not replicate the normal insulin profile

Fig. 37. Nateglinide principally targets postprandial glucose, and in previously treatment-naïve patients the combination of nateglinide and metformin is associated with significant reductions in both fasting and postprandial glucose. The effect on HbA₁c is additive with each agent causing a fall of around 1% as monotherapy, 2% in combination. Reproduced from Diabetes Care 2000;23:1660-5 with permission from the American Diabetes Association.

41

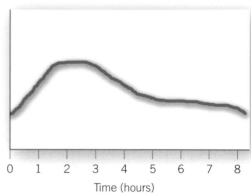

Plasma insulin

Time (hours)

❝ *Tight glycaemic control is difficult to achieve and there may be a price to pay from the point of view of increased risk of hypoglycaemia* **❞**

Fig. 38. A typical insulin profile after subcutaneous administration of soluble insulin. The graph shows a slow rise to maximum effect, a plateau effect and then fairly slow loss from the circulation.

consisting of a transient or meal-related component and a continuous or basal component. This has led to the development of a new range of insulin analogues or "designer insulins".

Rapid-acting insulin analogues

Standard subcutaneous insulin injection cannot mimic a normal daytime insulin profile. For example, after injection of soluble (regular) insulin there is an initial delay, loss of peak insulin response and a plateau effect with delayed loss of insulin from the circulation (Figure 38) – very different from normal physiology.[83] This means we advise our patients to inject insulin around 30 minutes before a meal and to eat snacks between meals to counter prolonged hyperinsulinaemia, which may lead to hypoglycaemia.

❝ *Standard subcutaneous insulin injection cannot mimic a normal daytime insulin profile* **❞**

The major problem with "rapid acting" insulins is they tend to form dimers and then hexamers subcutaneously, which must break back down to dimeric and monomeric units before they can be absorbed into the capillary circulation (Figure 39).[84] There are also problems with long-acting formulations, as will be discussed later.

To overcome some of these difficulties rapid-acting insulin analogues have been developed. One can simplistically define an insulin analogue as an insulin that has been modified in some way to retain its biological properties, but to have some advantage over standard insulins.

The ideal rapid-acting insulin would give peak plasma concentrations between 30 and 60 minutes after injection with a rapid return to basal levels by 180 minutes. Both Eli Lilly and NovoNordisk have developed insulin analogues to try to overcome some of these problems.

The approach taken by Eli Lilly was to switch the amino acids proline and lysine at positions 28 and 29 in the insulin B chain to lysine and proline (insulin lispro) (Figure 40).[83] This produces an insulin with much reduced tendency to self-association thereby preventing hexamer formation. The result is an insulin with a very rapid absorption, producing a fine peak and then rapid loss from the circulation, much more closely resembling a normal physiological insulin profile after a meal.

A similar approach was taken in developing the second of the rapid-acting insulin analogues, insulin aspart.[82]

More recently, premixed formulations of rapid-acting insulin analogues with intermediate-acting insulins have been developed. This is in recognition of the fact that although the rapid-acting analogues

66 The major problem with "rapid acting" insulins is they tend to form dimers and then hexamers subcutaneously 99

Fig. 39. Diagram illustrating the tendency of insulin molecules to form hexamers, which need to break down to dimers and monomers before they can be absorbed into the capillary circulation. This delays absorption into the capillaries even in patients administering so called "short-acting" insulin. Reproduced with permission from Pickup J, Williams G. Textbook of diabetes Vol 1. Oxford: Blackwell Publishing, 1991;375

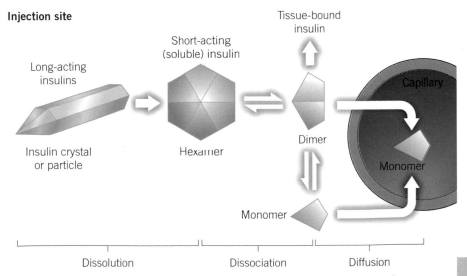

themselves are best used as part of a basal bolus regime (preprandial administration with a long-acting insulin at bedtime) many patients, particularly those with type 2 diabetes, prefer twice daily pre-mixed insulin formulations.

These rapid-acting analogues have been on the market for several years and their clinical characteristics compared with standard soluble insulins are now well described[85] as follows:

- Significant reduction in postprandial hyperglycaemia

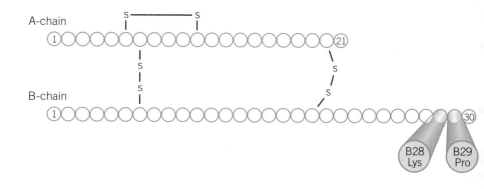

Fig. 40. The structure of insulin lispro. This differs from standard human insulin by switching of amino acids at position 28 and 29 in the insulin B chain.

- Reduction in hypoglycaemia, particularly nocturnal hypoglycaemia and severe hypoglycaemia in type 1 diabetes
- No significant improvement in HbA_{1c} in the large registration studies, but more focused studies have shown improvements compared with soluble insulin in certain situations.
- Improved patient satisfaction with the therapy, particularly because the insulin can be injected immediately before a meal, rather than waiting.

These insulins appear to have improved safety profiles for hypoglycaemia compared with standard soluble insulins, with no significant issues of immunogenicity.[86]

Structural homology to insulin-like growth factor-1 (IGF-1) has caused concerns that these analogues might have carcinogenic potential and/or might promote atheroma or microvascular progression.[83] This was a clear concern with one such analogue (Asp B10), which demonstrated increased incidence of mammary tumours in rodents over 1 year compared with standard insulins. These concerns have been allayed with the rapid-acting insulin analogues where there does not appear to be a problem.

Rapid-acting insulin analogues have been part of an ongoing evolution of insulin therapy. While they have not been a revolution, they do have some advantages over current soluble insulins.

There has been a long learning curve for these new insulins because they are not directly interchangeable with standard soluble insulins. To improve overall glycaemic control it is commonly necessary to increase the dose of basal insulin with a slight reduction in the preprandial dose of the insulin analogue compared with standard insulins. Trial data has also demonstrated that these agents are safer than soluble insulins during intense exercise, provided this is taken several hours after a meal, although the risk of hypoglycaemia if exercise is taken just after a meal is increased.

This type of insulin has also been particularly useful for children and people with significant psychiatric problems or senility, where it is difficult to predict how much will be eaten at mealtimes. The facility for postprandial administration is, therefore, particularly useful in this situation and provides at least as good diabetic control as that achieved with preprandial administration of standard insulins.

The full potential of rapid-acting insulin analogues has not been realized because of the lack of really good basal insulins with which to use them. This situation may be rectified with the new long-acting insulin analogues (see next section).

> **The ideal insulin would have a true 24-hour profile, a flattened action profile and a low risk of hypoglycaemia**

Basal insulin analogues

From the point of view of the basal component, the ideal insulin would have a true 24-hour profile, a flattened action profile and a low risk of hypoglycaemia.[87]

The problem with current basal insulins (isophane and lente) is they commonly do not produce a true 24-hour profile and there is large inter- and intra-patient variability of absorption from injection sites.[87] Isophane insulin, when injected at bedtime, tends to peak after 4 to 6 hours, which may produce nocturnal hypoglycaemia with a tendency to fasting hyperglycaemia in the morning. In practice, therefore, it is difficult to combine isophane insulin effectively with soluble or short-acting insulins within a basal bolus regime and patients are frequently exposed to nocturnal hypoglycaemia, morning fasting hyperglycaemia or both.

Another problem with traditional basal insulins is that rates of subcutaneous absorption vary between patients and differences in the site and depth of injection make it difficult to plan dosing accurately. In addition, re-suspension of isophane or lente insulin prior to injection from insulin pens is often inadequate with at least 20 inversions of

> **Another problem with traditional basal insulins is that rates of subcutaneous absorption vary between patients**

the pen needed to achieve proper mixing. In real life very few patients manage to achieve this.

Insulin glargine To try to overcome these limitations several basal insulin analogues have been or are being developed. The first, insulin glargine (Lantus, Aventis), has recently appeared on the market. It is produced through modification of human insulin by adding two arginine residues to the insulin B chain at the amino terminal end, and substituting a glycine for asparagine at position 21 of the A chain (Figure 41).[87]

As a result, the isoelectric point of the molecule is shifted from slightly acidic to near neutral pH. Insulin glargine is therefore present in solution in the slightly acidic conditions of the vial or cartridge but precipitates in the neutral pH of subcutaneous tissue. The result is an insulin with a delayed absorption, a late onset of action and prolonged duration of action.[88]

Subcutaneous injection of glargine produces a 24-hour profile and a low flat profile of systemic insulin exposure, which contrasts sharply with the peaking and declining profile and shorter duration of action observed with isophane insulin.

Compared with isophane insulin, glargine produces significantly greater reduction in fasting blood glucose when used as part of a basal bolus regimen in patients with type 1 diabetes.[89-92] Insulin glargine and isophane produce similar effects on HbA_{1c}, but the former is associated with significantly fewer episodes of nocturnal hypoglycaemia.

Studies in patients with type 2 diabetes have demonstrated that insulin glargine is at least as effective as isophane in achieving HbA_{1c} targets but with lower risks of nocturnal hypoglycaemia when used in combination with oral hypoglycaemic agents or with mealtime insulin (Figure 42).[93-97]

There are three potential advantages of insulin glargine over traditional basal insulins:

- Because insulin glargine has a flat action profile after injection, which more closely replicates the normal pattern of insulin secretion, it is less likely to cause hypoglycaemia, particularly nocturnal hypoglycaemia.
- It offers more reproducible glucose control, with less inter- and intra-patient variability, in part because of its preservation in solution.
- It gives improved convenience because of once daily dosing.
   This insulin has also recently had a licence extension to include children over 6 years old and flexible timing of injections (this means i

> **There is also evidence for improved treatment satisfaction and quality of life with insulin glargine**

can be given once daily in the morning or evening depending on patient preference).

There appear to be safety advantages of insulin glargine compared with traditional basal insulin from the point of view of hypoglycaemia. Concerns about its high affinity for the IGF-1 receptor[98] increasing the risk of retinopathy have been allayed[99] as have concerns regarding immunogenicity.

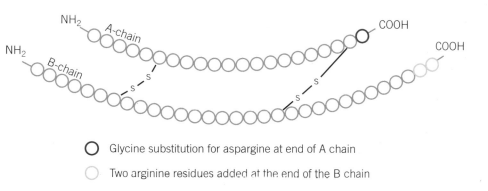

○ Glycine substitution for aspargine at end of A chain

○ Two arginine residues added at the end of the B chain

The advantages of insulin glargine over traditional insulins include a 24-hour profile, a flattened action profile with reduced risks of nocturnal hypoglycaemia and possibly less weight gain. There is also evidence for improved treatment satisfaction and quality of life. This insulin therefore appears to be an important addition to the range of insulins already available for both type 1 and type 2 diabetes.

Insulin detemir This is a new basal insulin analogue which should be licensed in 2004. It is soluble at neutral pH and designed to reversibly bind to albumin after subcutaneous injection.[100] It differs from human insulin by omission of the amino acid threonine at position 30 in the insulin B chain, and the attachment of a C14 fatty acid chain (myristic acid) to lysine at position 29 of the insulin B chain.[101] This side-chain also contributes to aggregation of insulin hexamers and delays its dissociation and absorption.[102]

After subcutaneous injection, this fatty acid side-chain rapidly binds to albumin both in the interstitial fluid and plasma with around 98% of the insulin being bound to albumin at any given time. The insulin then has to dissociate from albumin before it can exert its

Fig. 41. The structure of insulin glargine. The amino acid changes produce an insulin with a flattened action profile, 24-hour effect and with reduced risk of (nocturnal) hypoglycaemia compared with traditional basal insulins.

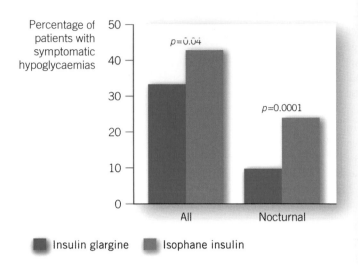

Percentage of patients with symptomatic hypoglycaemias

$p=0.04$

$p=0.0001$

All — Nocturnal

■ Insulin glargine ■ Isophane insulin

Fig. 42. There is significantly reduced risk of nocturnal hypoglycaemia in patients taking insulin glargine compared with isophane insulin when added to oral agents in patients with type 2 diabetes. Reproduced from Diabetes Care 2000; 238:1130-6 with permission from the American Diabetes Association.

biological effects. Such binding and dissociation occurs in subcutaneous tissue, interstitial tissue and in the blood stream. Monomers of insulin detemir then pass through the capillaries to reach the target tissues for binding with the insulin receptor.

The result is a basal insulin with prolonged action compared with isophane insulin, less inter- and intra-patient variability after subcutaneous injection and the potential for reduced risks of hypoglycaemia and weight gain.[103] The clinical trial programme so far in type 1 diabetes has demonstrated reduced risk of nocturnal hypoglycaemia and reduced fasting blood glucose compared with isophane insulin, but no overall improvement in glycaemic control based on HbA_{1c}.[103] Data on type 2 diabetes is accruing, but little has been published to date.

This new insulin represents an alternative approach to basal insulin therapy with the potential for similar benefits to insulin glargine, but by a different action. Further information is awaited but preliminary data looks promising.

Inhaled insulin
Several inhaled insulin formulations and delivery systems are being developed for type 1 and type 2 diabetes. This is not a new idea: in 1925, a German physician experimented with a nebulizer to deliver insulin![104] Lack of success until now is testimony to the fact that insulin is still, more than 80 years after its discovery, given by subcutaneous injection.

The large surface area and high permeability of the lung make it an ideal delivery route for insulin.[105] There is little absorption of insulin particles in the bronchi and it is thought these molecules are absorbed into the lungs by transcytosis across the alveolar epithelial cells and the alveolar capillary endothelial cells. The insulin then diffuses into the blood stream to exert its biological effect.

The first preparation likely to be on the market was developed by Inhaled Therapeutic Systems, and Pfizer and Aventis are currently conducting phase 3 clinical trials.[106] The system delivers a fine powder formulation of short-acting human insulin to the lung in a reproducible manner.

The delivery device is similar to a portable nebulizer with a chamber to capture a standing cloud of fine insulin particles. A blister pack containing a range of insulin doses is inserted into the inhaler, a pneumatic mechanism punctures the blister packs inside the inhaler and the insulin particles are released into the air chamber and then slowly inhaled by the patient with one deep breath.

Both slow-release and fast-acting insulin formulations for inhalation are also being tested by Alkermes using the AIR delivery system, which administers porous particles of 10-20mm diameter.[106] The device aerosotizes the particles from blister packs and is breath activated.

There are several other devices in development, including Aradigm's AERx drug delivery system, AeroGen's liquid insulin delivery and the Pharmaceutical Discovery Corporation's Technosphere technology.[106]

Whatever system is used, inhaled insulin has a more rapid onset of action than subcutaneously injected insulin and is likely to be particularly useful for postprandial blood glucose control.[106]

Using the Pfizer/Aventis insulin dry powder pulmonary inhaler in a three-way crossover study, inhaled insulin had a faster onset of action than regular insulin with an offset of action between that of insulin lispro (rapid-acting insulin analogue) and regular insulin.[107] This was in healthy male volunteers, but comparisons have also been made in patients with type 2 diabetes.[108] In this group the pharma-cokinetic profile of inhaled insulin was similar to subcutaneous insulin, again suggesting inhaled insulin is appropriate for pre-meal dosing.

Similar properties have been ascribed to AERx in patients with type 1 diabetes compared with subcutaneous insulin.[109]

For patients with type 2 diabetes, inadequately controlled on oral agents, adding inhaled insulin preprandially resulted in significantly greater reductions in HbA_{1c} than oral therapy alone.[110]

> **The large surface area and high permeability of the lung make it an ideal delivery route for insulin**

> **Inhaled insulin is likely to be particularly useful for postprandial blood glucose control**

49

In an open-label study of 73 patients with type 1 diabetes, patients were given their usual daily insulin regimen of two to three injections or pre-meal inhaled insulin, plus a bedtime ultra lente injection.[111] There was no significant difference in glycaemic control (fasting or postprandial glucose concentrations) after 12 weeks (Figure 43).

"Studies in type 2 diabetes have demonstrated stable HbA_{1c} with inhaled insulin"

Studies in type 2 diabetes with patient follow-up after 2 years have demonstrated stable HbA_{1c} with inhaled insulin.[112]

To date, the limited clinical trial data demonstrates significantly greater improvement in treatment satisfaction for patients with type 1 or type 2 diabetes when comparing inhaled insulin with standard subcutaneous injections or with oral agents alone.[111-113]

Fig. 43. Concentration of HbA_{1c} in blood during 12-week treatment period comparing subcutaneous and inhaled insulin. The response of HbA_{1c} to treatment did not vary between the two groups. Reproduced from Skyler JS. Efficacy of inhaled insulin in type 1 diabetes mellitus: a randomised proof-of-concept study. Lancet 2001;357:331-5 with permission from Elsevier.

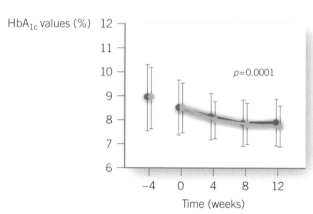

The limited data available also suggests inhaled dry powder insulin is well tolerated. These studies have shown no increased incidence of hypoglycaemia compared with subcutaneous insulin.

A major issue is whether long-term inhalation of insulin might have deleterious effects on the lung alveoli and the bronchial tree. This clearly needs intense study, but to date no major issues have arisen.

The limited data so far suggests inhaled insulin is as effective and well tolerated as subcutaneous insulin in both type 1 and type 2 diabetes. There appears to be improved patient satisfaction, perhaps not surprising! More studies are needed to confirm long-term efficacy to compare the different approaches to find the relative place in practice and provide long-term safety data.

One hopes that inhaled insulin might improve patient compliance and might be particularly important in facilitating earlier initiation of insulin treatment in patients with type 2 diabetes – too often delayed with resulting negative consequences on general health, well-being and perhaps development of long-term complications.

One issue is that to date only rapid-acting inhaled insulin formulations have been tested. Until long-acting formulations are developed, inhaled insulin will not totally abolish the need for subcutaneous injections (certainly in people with type 1 diabetes) but will reduce the number required.

Given the increasing emphasis on intensive diabetes treatment and the very good evidence that such treatment will help prevent long-term complications in the growing number of patients with type 2 diabetes, one can predict there will be an increasingly important role for novel drug delivery systems for insulin in the management of diabetes.

> *There will be an increasingly important role for novel drug delivery systems for insulin*

Dyslipidaemia

Clinical trials have shown profound benefits in terms of cardiovascular morbidity and mortality from HMG-CoA reductase inhibitors (statins). The benefits relate, at least in part, to cholesterol lowering, but statins may have other effects, such as reducing inflammation, which could also contribute to risk reduction.

Published targets include reduction of total cholesterol to less than 5mmol/l and LDL to less than 3mmol/l but, as already described, results from the Heart Protection Study[50] make this concept redundant. Many specialists believe that as type 2 diabetes is a cardiovascular disease, the approach to management should include "statins for all". This has, in part, been recognized by the recent guidance from the National Institute for Clinical Excellence,[33] which recommends statin treatment for patients with diabetes where 10-year coronary heart disease risk is greater than 15% (in practice, most people with type 2 diabetes).

Given that the typical dyslipidaemia of type 2 diabetes is low HDL and raised triglycerides, there may also be a significant role for fibrates and there is preliminary evidence supporting this.[114] For patients with normal total cholesterol but low HDL and raised triglycerides a fibrate may be a suitable first-line treatment. For the (majority) of patients where statins are indicated but who have low HDL and raised triglycerides a combination of statin and fibrate may be particularly efficacious, but may also be associated with increased risk of side-effects.

> *The National Institute of Clinical Excellence recommends statin treatment for patients with diabetes where 10-year CHD risk is greater than 15%*

HMG-CoA reductase inhibitors (statins)

Statins were originally derived from fungal metabolites and are competitive inhibitors of HMG-CoA reductase, this enzyme being involved in the rate-limiting step in cholesterol biosythesis: conversion of HMG-CoA to mevalonate.[115]

> *Maximum effect with statins is achieved by giving the drug at bedtime as the majority of hepatic cholesterol biosynthesis occurs overnight*

Statins have an open-ring structure similar to the HMG-CoA molecule leading to competition for the active site of the enzyme. Statins therefore cause a fall in hepatic cholesterol synthesis, with up-regulation of LDL receptors and a fall in plasma LDL concentrations.

They are effective in lowering LDL cholesterol in a dose-dependent manner by up to 40% and maximum effect is achieved by giving the drug at bedtime as the majority of hepatic cholesterol biosynthesis occurs overnight. Tolerability is relatively good, although liver function tests and plasma creatinine kinase levels should be measured before starting therapy and intermittently thereafter.

At the time of writing there are four statins available in the UK. These include atorvastatin, fluvastatin, pravastatin and simvastatin. Recently cerivastatin has been withdrawn because of increased incidence of rhabdomyolysis, particularly in association with the fibrate gemfibrozil. The other statins have a much lower incidence of these problems and there were no incidences of fatal rhabdomyolysis in more than 30,000 patients participating in the large statin trials.

Recently even more potent statins ("super statins") have been developed. The first – rosuvastatin – is licensed for use.

"Super statins"

A new generation of statins has recently been introduced onto the market. They have demonstrated potency both *in vitro* and *in vivo* greater than with traditional statins (Figure 44).

The first, rosuvastatin (Crestor, Astra Zeneca), is relatively hydrophilic and, unlike several other statins, not metabolized by the cytochrome CYP450 3A4 enzyme.[115] It should not interact significantly with drugs that are metabolized by this route, thereby offering potential safety advantages.

Early clinical studies have shown that rosuvastatin improves total cholesterol, LDL cholesterol and raises HDL cholesterol with beneficial effects on triglycerides. The later Clinical Trials Programme has demonstrated that in patients with primary hypercholesterolaemia, 80mg of rosuvastatin is associated with a 65% reduction in LDL cholesterol compared with baseline.[116]

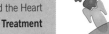

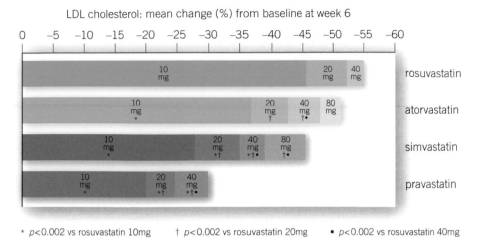

LDL cholesterol: mean change (%) from baseline at week 6

* p<0.002 vs rosuvastatin 10mg   † p<0.002 vs rosuvastatin 20mg   • p<0.002 vs rosuvastatin 40mg

Fig. 44. The greater potency of rosuvastatin compared with other statins at an equivalent dosage. Reproduced from J Am Coll Cardiol 2003;41(in press) with permission from The American College of Cardiology Foundation.

Rosuvastatin also compares favourably with the next most powerful statin, atorvastatin (Figure 45). Over 12 weeks, patients with hypercholesterolaemia receiving 5mg or 10mg of rosuvastatin had a reduction in LDL cholesterol of 40% and 43% respectively, compared with a 35% reduction in patients receiving atorvastatin at 10mg once daily.[117] Both doses of rosuvastatin were associated with increased HDL cholesterol greater than that seen with atorvastatin (13% versus 8%).

Other comparisons have shown that in patients with dyslipidaemia 10mg of rosuvastatin is associated with significantly greater reductions in LDL cholesterol than with atorvastatin 10mg, simvastatin 20mg and pravastatin 20mg.[117,118]

Clinical trial data for rosuvastatin suggest good toleration and a safety profile similar to other statins. Liver function disturbance was seen in one in 200 patients and evidence of myopathy in one in 500 (in those patients taking the highest dose of rosuvastatin). All problems resolved after stopping the drug.

Cholesterol absorption inhibitors
A new class of agents has recently been developed for managing dyslipidaemia. The first of which – ezetimibe or ezetrol (Merck Sharp and Dohme Ltd/Schering-Plough Ltd) – has recently been licensed (Figure 46).

❝ The new generation of super statins have demonstrated potency greater than with traditional statins ❞

53

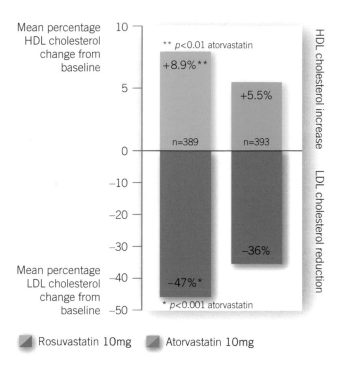

Mean percentage HDL cholesterol change from baseline

** *p<0.01* atorvastatin

+8.9%**

+5.5%

n=389   n=393

HDL cholesterol increase

LDL cholesterol reduction

Mean percentage LDL cholesterol change from baseline

−47%*

−36%

* *p<0.001* atorvastatin

Rosuvastatin 10mg   Atorvastatin 10mg

Fig. 45. Improvement in LDL cholesterol and HDL cholesterol with rosuvastatin compared with atorvastatin.
Reproduced from Am J Cardiol 2003;91(suppl):3C-10C with permission from Excerpta Medica Inc.

To date, the management of dyslipidaemia has relied primarily on monotherapy with statins to lower total and LDL cholesterol, with some reported beneficial effects on triglycerides. Fibrates have been reserved for patients with low HDL cholesterol and raised triglycerides and can be used in combination with statins, although this combination may increase the risk of side-effects, including myalgic symptoms and occasionally rhabdomyolysis.

Although the evidence base for statins is extremely strong with regard to reducing cardiovascular morbidity and mortality, a significant percentage of patients with dyslipidaemia do not respond optimally to this treatment. This may include a group of patients who show elevated intestinal absorption of dietary cholesterol, rather than increased cholesterol synthesis.

Mechanism of action of cholesterol absorption inhibitors
Cholesterol absorption is a complex and multifaceted process and involves incorporation into mixed micelles, together with bile salts and plant sterols.[119] This is then endocytosed by intestinal mucosa cells and

transported to the endoplasmic reticulum for incorporation into chylomicrons.

The plant sterols and part of the endocytosed cholesterol is re-secreted back into the lumen of the intestine by retro-endocytosis. The ABC transporter (ABCA1) is required for this re-secretion.

The cholesterol absorption inhibitor ezetimibe inhibits the uptake of micellar sterols by the intestine and thereby lowers the absorption of cholesterol and plant sterol simultaneously (Figure 47). In theory, combining ezetimibe with a statin will simultaneously decrease cholesterol absorption and synthesis thereby having great therapeutic potential for patients hyperabsorbing cholesterol.

66 The cholesterol absorption inhibitor ezetimibe inhibits the uptake of micellar sterols by the intestine 99

Clinical studies

The efficacy and safety of ezetimibe monotherapy has been demonstrated in four large placebo-controlled, double-blind, studies.[120-122] Patients with primary hypercholesterolaemia were enrolled and pooled results from phase 3 trials have shown that 10mg ezetimibe significantly reduces LDL cholesterol by 17% and increases HDL cholesterol by 1%, with decreased triglycerides of 4%, compared with placebo. This is accompanied by excellent tolerability and safety profiles.

A particularly difficult group of patients includes those with homozygous familial hypercholesterolaemia. In patients refractory to

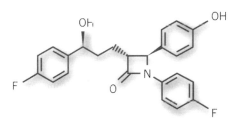

Fig. 46. Structure of ezetimibe. Ezetimibe is a potent and specific inhibitor of dietary and biliary cholesterol absorption.

statins, a recent study showed that addition of ezetimibe 10mg daily to atorvastatin or simvastatin 80mg daily resulted in an extra 20% decrease in LDL cholesterol.[123]

Several studies have shown that ezetimibe can be co-administered with statins to provide complimentary synergistic effects in patients with hypercholesterolaemia (Figures 48 and 49). Significant reductions in LDL cholesterol and triglycerides and increases in HDL levels have

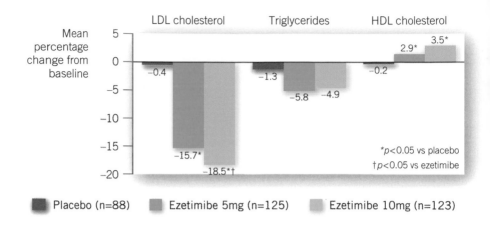

Placebo (n=88)   Ezetimibe 5mg (n=125)   Ezetimibe 10mg (n=123)

Fig. 47. Effects of ezetimibe on LDL cholesterol, triglyceride, and HDL cholesterol. Pooled phase II monotherapy results. Demonstrated reduction in LDL cholesterol of around 18 per cent with this therapy at the 10mg recommended dose together with improvement in HDL cholesterol. Reproduced from J Am Coll Cardiol 2000;35(suppl A):257A with permission from The American College of Cardiology Foundation.

been demonstrated using this combination when compared with either statin alone.[124-126]

Place of ezetimibe in therapy

Achieving equivalent reductions of LDL cholesterol seen with ezetimibe/statin combination compared with a statin alone frequently means increasing to maximum does of statin. This often requires dose titration, is time consuming and may increase the risk of liver and muscle toxicity. In addition, each doubling of statin dose may produce only a 6% further reduction in LDL cholesterol.

Another approach is to co-administer ezetimibe and a low-dose statin. This produces similar benefits to the lipid profiles as high-dose statins and is extremely well tolerated.

A further possibility is co-administration of ezetimibe with a fibrate. This might be particularly beneficial in patients with combined dyslipidaemia or type 2 diabetes (although this is not currently a licensed indication). In a study of ezetimibe plus fenofibrate[127] there was no evidence of pharmacodynamic or pharmacokinetic interactions and in this healthy group there was a greater than 22% reduction in LDL cholesterol after 2 weeks of combination treatment compared with fibrate alone.

Conclusions

Cholesterol absorption inhibitors represent a new approach to lipid management. Statins mainly affect cholesterol synthesis in the liver, whereas ezetimibe mainly affects cholesterol absorption from the gut. The effects on total and LDL cholesterol are, therefore, additive with

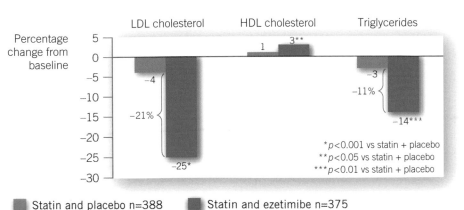

Statin and placebo n=388   Statin and ezetimibe n=375

the added bonus of possible increase in HDL and reduction in triglycerides.

Given the excellent evidence base for statins in reducing cardio-vascular morbidity and mortality, the main place for these new agents will be in combination therapy. This will allow lower doses of statins to be used, thereby reducing the risk of side-effects. They may also have a role in patients who cannot tolerate statins and in situations where powerful drug effects in combination with

Fig. 48. Effect of ezetimibe on lipid levels when added to ongoing statin therapy. Reproduced from Am J Cardiol 2002;90:1084-1091 with permission from Excerpta Medica Inc.

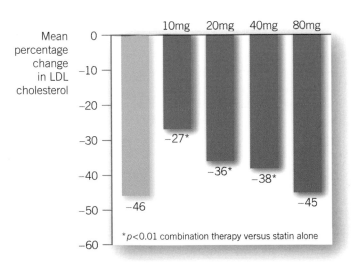

Fig. 49. Ezetimibe and simvastatin study: efficacy on LDL cholesterol. Reproduced from Am J Cardiol 2002 (Abstract) with permission from Excerpta Medica Inc.

Ezetimibe (10mg) + simvastatin (10mg)   Simvastatin

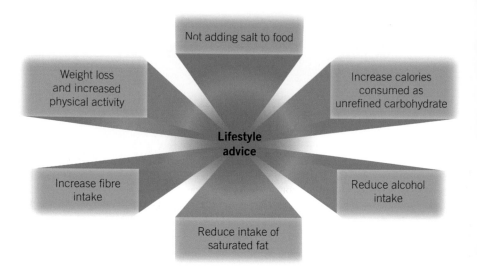

Fig. 50. Lifestyle advice to reduce blood pressure in patients with type 2 diabetes.

high-dose statins are needed, such as in patients with familial hypercholesterolaemia.

New agents for bile acid sequestration
The first of these new drugs likely to appear on the market is colesevelan hydrochloride (Cholestagel, Genzyme), which is a non-absorbed lipid-lowering agent specifically engineered to efficiently bind bile acids in the intestine thereby impeding absorption. Such bile sequestration results in increased clearance of LDL cholesterol.

Clinical trial data have demonstrated significant reductions in LDL cholesterol with some increase in HDL cholesterol. Colesevelan is currently licensed in the US for combination with statins to help reach target, and can also be used as monotherapy in patients who are statin intolerant. The LDL-lowering effect is similar to that achieved with the cholesterol absorption inhibitors: around 15% to 18%.

The side-effect profile includes gastrointestinal disturbance in a relatively small percentage of patients. Liver function monitoring is not required when used as monotherapy.

The product is expected to be launched in Europe some time in 2004.

> **❝ Colesevelan is a non-absorbed lipid-lowering agent specifically engineered to efficiently bind bile acids in the intestine ❞**

Aspirin

British Hypertension Society guidelines suggest diabetic patients with hypertension and a 10-year coronary heart disease risk greater than 15% should be on low-dose (75mg once daily) aspirin once the blood pressure is controlled.[29]

It is the authors' practice to prescribe 75mg aspirin routinely to all diabetic patients with another cardiovascular risk factor and/or 10-year coronary heart disease risk greater than 15%, provided there is no contraindication.

Hypertension

The benefits of tight blood pressure control have been clearly demonstrated and are profound. For diabetic patients with mild-to-moderate hypertension (systolic 140mmHg to 160mmHg and/or diastolic 90mmHg to 100mmHg), non-pharmacological therapy might be a first approach but should not be too prolonged.

Lifestyle advice should include the measures shown in Figure 50. These measures can result in significant blood pressure reduction, but in most cases combination with antihypertensive agents will be necessary to get down to the current much tighter targets.

Early intervention is particularly required in patients with a past history of cardiovascular disease, and in those with a high cardiovascular risk (greater than 15% over 10 years – in practice most diabetic patients), or if there is evidence of end-organ damage such as:

- left ventricular hypertrophy
- nephropathy
- renal impairment
- hypertensive retinopathy.

For type 1 diabetic patients, who are often thin, early antihypertensive treatment may be especially relevant, particularly with an ACE inhibitor.

Drug therapy for managing hypertension in diabetes may present some special difficulties in diabetic patients because of:

- metabolic side-effects that could provoke dyslipidaemia, deterioration in diabetic control and electrolyte imbalance
- certain complications, particularly autonomic neuropathy, peripheral vascular disease and renal impairment may cause intolerance or frank contraindication to some antihypertensives
- achieving target blood pressure with single agents is not possible in most diabetic patients. This means using several drugs from different antihypertensive classes, which may cause concern about drug interactions, patient compliance and cost.

> ❝ *For diabetic patients with mild-to-moderate hypertension non-pharmacological therapy might be a first approach but should not be too prolonged* ❞

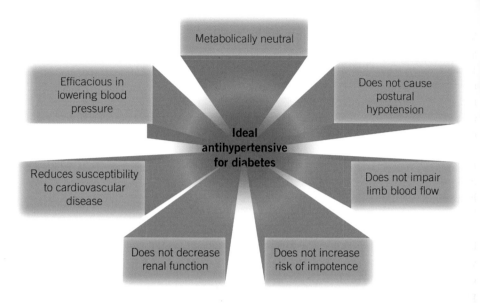

The ideal drug for the diabetic patient should have the properties shown in Figure 51. The major drug classes include thiazide diuretics, beta blockers, specific alpha blockers, calcium channel blockers and renin-angiotensin system inhibitors.

Thiazides and beta-blockers[128]

These drugs are efficacious in lowering blood pressure, cheap, suitable for once daily dosing with evidence of cardiovascular protection. Diuretics have been shown to reduce the incidence of stroke, heart failure and risk of cardiovascular disease, and beta blockers are cardio-protective particularly post-myocardial infarction. In the UKPDS hypertension trial,[39] beta blockade was associated with reduced cardio-vascular risk and mortality in patients with type 2 diabetes. They are also useful with coincident angina.

These drug classes gained a bad name because of putative meta-bolic side-effects (Figure 52), but many early studies used doses of thi-azides, in particular, much higher than required for maximum blood pressure lowering. Such side-effects included deterioration in gly-caemia, worsening dyslipidaemia, erectile dysfunction and, in the case of beta blockers, masking the warning symptoms of hypoglycaemia.

Thiazides and beta blockers are a useful part of the armamentar-ium of drugs to manage hypertension in diabetes, and are commonly used as second- or third-line agents combined with more modern drugs.

" Thiazides and beta blockers are a useful part of the armamentarium of drugs to manage hypertension in diabetes "

Thiazide-like diuretics

The only such drug in common use is indapamide, which is now available also in a slow-release formulation (Natrilix SR 1.5mg , Servier Laboratories). This drug is derived from a sulphonamide and is pharmacologically related to thiazide diuretics. Its antihypertensive effect is linked to improved arterial compliance and a reduction in arteriolar and total peripheral resistance. It also acts on the kidney resulting in diuresis, though less marked than that seen with traditional thiazides.

There is evidence for metabolic neutrality, which makes it particularly suitable for certain patients, such as those with type 2 diabetes, dyslipidaemia and renal insufficiency.[129] The slow-release formulation has a 24-hour antihypertensive effect equivalent to that seen with long-acting calcium channel blockers and ACE inhibitors.[130-132]

Although indapamide has been around for many years, there has been much recent interest after trial data demonstrated reduced left ventricular hypertrophy greater than that seen with the ACE inhibitor enalapril, an effect in part independent of blood pressure lowering and possibly a result of a direct and progressive effect on the heart.[132] In addition, this agent is associated with a significant reduction in albumin excretion rate in patients with type 2 diabetes and microalbuminuria, similar in magnitude to that seen with ACE inhibitors.[133,134]

In the PROGRESS study,[135] over 6000 patients with a previous history of stroke or transient ischaemic attack were randomized to receive an ACE inhibitor (perindopril) or placebo. Indapamide and

Fig. 52. Metabolic profiles of different antihypertensive drug classes. Note that both beta blockers and, in particular, thiazides are very useful antihypertensives in combination. Deleterious metabolic side-effects are more likely at higher doses, especially with thiazides. Combination treatment is normally required to achieve target blood pressure.

	Beta blockers	Thiazides	Alpha blockers	Calcium channel blockers	ACE I	AIIA
Glycaemia	↑	↑	-	-	-	-
Dyslipidaemia	↑	↑	-	-	-	-
Insulin resistance	↑	↑	(↓)	-	(↓)	(↓)
Electrolyte imbalance	-	Low K⁺	-	-	-	-
Erectile dysfunction	↑	↑	-	-	-	-

- Neutral ↑ Deterioration (↓) Borderline improvement
ACE I = ACE inhibitors AIIA = angiotensin II receptor antagonists

perindopril were co-administered to the active group. The patients, who could be hypertensive or normotensive, were followed up over four years. Active treatment reduced relative risk of stroke by 28% and the risk of total major vascular events by 25%. This improvement was particularly marked when an ACE inhibitor and indapamide were used, with an overall stroke risk reduction of 43% irrespective of whether the patient was hypertensive or normotensive.

The potential value of thiazide or thiazide-like approach to hypertension management was also emphasized by the Antihypertensive and Lipid Lowering Treatment to prevent Heart Attack Trial (ALLHAT).[136] This was a randomized, double-blind, active-controlled, clinical trial conducted between February 1994 and March 2002. The objective was to determine whether treatment with a calcium channel blocker or an ACE inhibitor lowered the incidence of coronary heart disease or other cardiovascular disease versus treatment with a thiazide diuretic. The drugs used were amlodipine, lisinopril and chlorthalidone.

The primary outcome was combined fatal coronary heart disease or non-fatal myocardial infarction analysed by intention to treat. Secondary outcomes were all-cause mortality/combined coronary heart disease and combined cardiovascular disease.

Mean follow up was 4.9 years and there was no difference between the treatments for the primary outcome. In addition, all-cause mortality did not differ between the groups. One can conclude that thiazide-type diuretics are at least as good as ACE inhibitors or calcium channel blockers in the management of hypertension. They are certainly reasonable first-line treatments in this context, although as already discussed the vast majority of diabetic patients with hypertension will require combination antihypertensive therapy.

> ❝ *Thiazide-type diuretics are certainly reasonable first-line treatments in the management of hypertension* ❞

Calcium channel blockers[128]

These can be divided into dihydropyridine and non-dihydropyridine classes. The latter have a longer elimination half-life and can be used for once daily dosing. These agents:

- have peripheral vasodilating properties and are antianginal, antiarrhythmic and cardioprotective
- have a neutral metabolic profile
- improve coronary blood flow and reduce cardiac afterload thereby reducing the work of the heart
- regress left ventricular hypertrophy.

They are a suitable antihypertensive treatment for diabetic patients with a good safety profile, but have a high incidence of minor side-effects such as ankle oedema and flushing of the face.

Specific alpha blockers[128]

These agents, such as doxazosin, are less likely to cause some of the problems reported with the older alpha blockers such as prazosin, which sometimes caused first-dose hypotension and postural hypotension. Some of their properties are shown in Figure 53.

Unfortunately, there is no long-term outcome data. Their use was being studied in the Antihypertensive and Lipid Lowering treatment to prevent Heart Attack Trial (ALLHAT),[137] but a recent interim analysis has resulted in the doxazosin group being discontinued because the treatment was associated with a 25% increase in relative risk of combined cardiovascular end points compared with thiazides. This mainly related to heart failure and stroke but with no evidence of increased mortality.

> *Specific alpha blockers are less likely to cause some of the problems reported with the older alpha blockers*

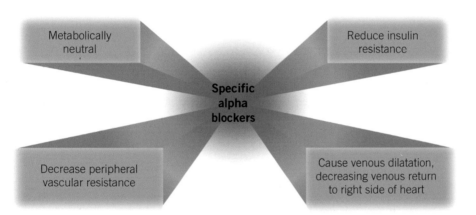

Fig. 53. Properties of specific alpha blockers.

These agents are not normally recommended first line for hypertension in diabetes, but can be very useful in combination with other classes of antihypertensives.

Inhibitors of the renin-angiotensin system

These agents have gained particular interest recently years. There are two major classes: angiotensin converting enzyme (ACE) inhibitors and angiotensin II receptor antagonists.

ACE inhibitors

It is not surprising these drugs reduce blood pressure because the renin-angiotensin system is intimately concerned with blood pressure

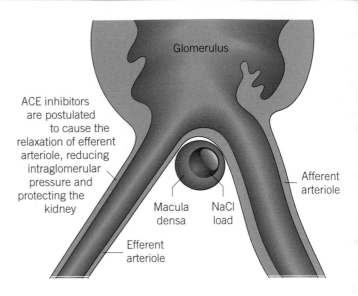

Glomerulus

ACE inhibitors
are postulated
to cause the
relaxation of efferent
arteriole, reducing
intraglomerular
pressure and
protecting the
kidney

Macula
densa

NaCl
load

Afferent
arteriole

Efferent
arteriole

Fig. 54. Putative mechanisms for the reno-protective effects of ACE inhibitors.

control and fluid and electrolyte balance (Figure 54).[138] ACE inhibitors prevent conversion of inactive angiotensin I to the active component angiotensin II resulting in:

- reduction of sympathetic tone
- decrease in elevated systemic vascular resistance
- enhanced perfusion of the heart and kidneys. Studies[128] have shown:
- efficacy in lowering blood pressure
- reversal of left ventricular hypertrophy
- benefit in patients with congestive heart failure reducing both morbidity and mortality
- metabolic neutrality
- possible reduced risk of type 2 diabetes in those at high risk.

66 ACE inhibitors have been shown to have renoprotective effects with some evidence also for protection of the retina 99

ACE inhibitors have been shown to have renoprotective effects with some evidence also for protection of the retina.[128] Very tight blood pressure control is the most important aspect of management of both incipient and overt diabetic nephropathy.[30] In patients with type 1 diabetes ACE inhibitors have been shown to slow the progression of overt diabetic renal disease and reduce mortality. In type 2 diabetes there is evidence for reduction in albumin excretion rate, although little hard end-point data is available.

The recently published Heart Outcomes Prevention Evaluation (HOPE) study examined the incidence of cardiovascular end points and mortality in people at high risk of cardiovascular disease.[44] Around 3500 of the 9500 patients were diabetic and had either a previous history of cardiovascular disease or one other cardiovascular risk factor. Patients were randomized to receive the ACE inhibitor ramipril or placebo and both groups could have any other therapy, including anti-hypertensives, except for inhibitors of the renin–angiotensin system.

There was a clear split in survival curves in favour of ACE inhibition (Figure 55) with highly significant reduction in:

- the primary composite end point of death, myocardial infarction and stroke (25%)
- overall mortality (24%)
- myocardial infarction (22%)
- stroke (33%)
- transient ischaemic attack and cardiovascular death (37%).

The study was terminated early at 4 years and, indeed, benefit was noted between 6 and 8 months after randomization.

This study is supported by a 6-year randomized trial (Captopril Prevention Project) comparing ACE inhibition with conventional therapy (beta blocker or thiazide) in terms of cardiovascular end points and mortality in hypertensive patients.[43] In almost 600 diabetic patients there was no significant difference in blood pressure, but the group who received the ACE inhibitor showed significant reductions in myocardial infarction (34%) and all cardiac events (67%).

Further support for the benefits of ACE inhibition comes from the PROGRESS study,[135] which randomized over 6000 individuals with a previous history of stroke or transient ischaemic attack into active ACE inhibition (perindopril) with or without indapamide versus

Fig. 55. Relative risk reduction in primary end points in favour of ACE inhibition in the HOPE study.
Reproduced from Results of the HOPE study and MICRO-HOPE sub-study. Lancet 2000;355:253-9 with permission from Elsevier.

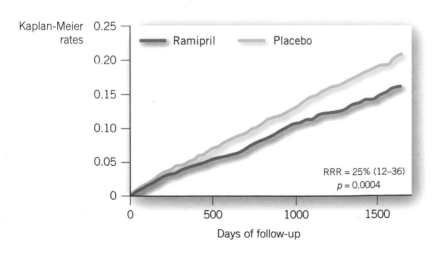

placebo groups. Patients could be hypertensive or normotensive and over 4 years of follow up, active treatment reduced relative risk of further stroke by 28% (Figure 56) and the risk of total major vascular events by 25%. Where the combination of ACE inhibition and indapamide was used, overall stroke risk was reduced by 43%. Similar risk reduction was seen in both hypertensive and normotensive individuals.

ACE inhibitors may also be useful in combination with diuretics in the management of heart failure. There is also evidence of a reduction in mortality in patients following a myocardial infarction, and studies have demonstrated regression of structural changes in left ventricular hypertrophy.[128]

They have a good tolerability profile, although chronic cough may lead to discontinuation in around 10% of patients. First-dose hypotension may also occur but this is rare. It is wise, however, to start ACE inhibitors at the lowest dose and to take the first dose just before bedtime. Discontinuation of diuretics for a few days before and just after starting an ACE inhibitor also reduces risks.

They should not be used in the presence of renal artery stenosis because this may be associated with deterioration of renal function. Such problems are rare even in elderly type 2 diabetic patients, but it is still wise to check creatinine 7 to 10 days after starting an ACE inhibitor and after each dose increase.

Fig. 56. PROGRESS study: cumulative incidence of stroke among participants assigned active treatment and those assigned placebo. Reproduced from PROGRESS Collaborative Group. Lancet 2001;358:1033-41 with permission from Elsevier.

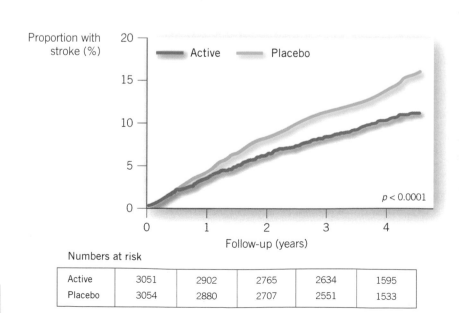

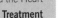

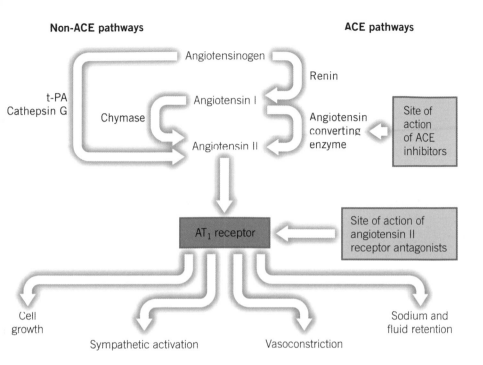

Fig. 57. The renin-angiotensin system and site of action of ACE inhibitors and angiotensin II receptor antagonists.

To summarize, ACE inhibitors are now important first-line treatments for managing hypertension in diabetes because they are:

- efficacious
- have a good tolerability profile
- metabolically neutral
- suitable for a wide range of patients and they can be used in combination with any drug from another antihypertensive class
- cardiac and renal protective.

Angiotensin II receptor antagonists

These agents also inhibit the renin-angiotensin system, but by blocking the effect of angiotensin II at the (type 1) receptor site (Figure 57).[139]

Angiotensin II receptor antagonists:

- are as efficacious as ACE inhibitors
- do not normally cause chronic cough
- are metabolically neutral
- are as good as ACE inhibitors in delaying progression of renal injury in animal models of disease[140]
- show renal protection, according to small clinical studies.[141]

Reproduced from Clinical Management of Hypertension. Barnett AH (ed). London: Martin Dunitz, 2002, p52 with permission from Thompson Publishing Services.

Recently, several trials in diabetic patients have extolled the benefits of angiotensin II receptor antagonists, from the point of view of renal protection (note also that diabetic renal disease is associated with massively increased risk of cardiovascular disease). Two studies have involved irbesartan and a third study involved losartan.

The first, IRMA2, looked at the effect of irbesartan on microalbuminuria in hypertensive type 2 diabetic patients.[142] Almost 600 patients with type 2 diabetes, hypertension and microalbuminuria, with normal creatinine, were studied. They were randomly assigned to

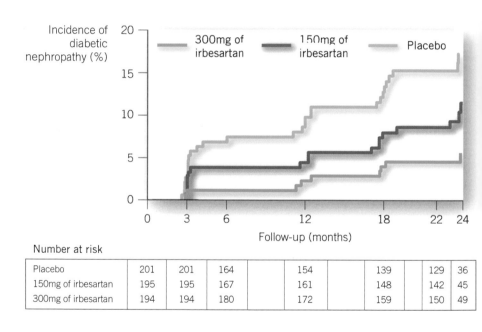

Number at risk							
Placebo	201	201	164	154	139	129	36
150mg of irbesartan	195	195	167	161	148	142	45
300mg of irbesartan	194	194	180	172	159	150	49

Fig. 58. The 70% risk reduction in hypertensive type 2 diabetic patients of progressing from microalbuminuria to overt nephropathy in favour of irbesartan compared with placebo. Reproduced from Parving H-H et al. The Effect of Irbesartan on the Development of Diabetic Nephropathy in Patients. N Engl J Med 2001;345:870-8. Copyright 2001 Massachusetts Medical Society. All rights reserved.

irbesartan 150mg once daily, 300mg once daily or to placebo. The primary outcome was time to onset of diabetic nephropathy defined by an albumin excretion rate higher than 200µg/min and at least 30% higher than baseline. The 300mg group showed a significant risk reduction of 70% compared with placebo of progression to overt nephropathy (p<0.001) (Figure 58). For the lower-dose group the relative risk reduction was 39% compared with control (p=0.08).

The second study (IDNT) was a 3-year trial, which studied more than 1700 hypertensive type 2 diabetic patients comparing irbesartan and the calcium channel blocker amlodipine versus placebo.[143] Other antihypertensives could be used to treat blood pressure. At randomization the patients had normal or raised creatinine and significant proteinuria.

The primary outcome was time to a composite end point consisting of a doubling of the baseline creatinine level, end-stage renal disease and death. For the primary end point the irbesartan group

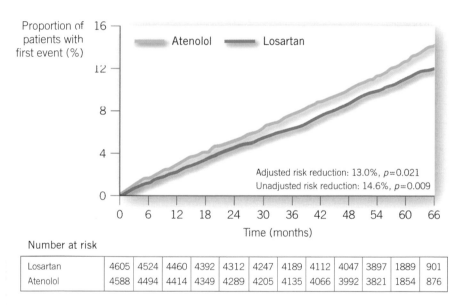

Proportion of patients with first event (%)

Adjusted risk reduction: 13.0%, $p=0.021$
Unadjusted risk reduction: 14.6%, $p=0.009$

Time (months)

Number at risk

	0	6	12	18	24	30	36	42	48	54	60	66
Losartan	4605	4524	4460	4392	4312	4247	4189	4112	4047	3897	1889	901
Atenolol	4588	4494	4414	4349	4289	4205	4135	4066	3992	3821	1854	876

Fig. 59. Adjusted and unadjusted risk reduction of around 14% in primary composite end point in the LIFE study in favour of losartan compared with atenolol. Reproduced from Dahlof B et al. Cardiovascular morbidity and mortality in the Losartan Intervention For Endpoint reduction in hypertension study (LIFE): a randomised trial against atenolol. Lancet 2002;359:995-1010 with permission from Elsevier.

showed a relative risk reduction of 20% compared with placebo (p=0.02) and 23% compared with the amlodipine group (p=0.006).

A similar trial in diabetic nephropathy (RENAAL) compared losartan 50-100mg with placebo in hypertensive type 2 diabetic patients with proteinuria.[144] The relative risk reduction for the primary composite end point was significant at 16% compared with control (p=0.02).

Unfortunately none of these trials was powered to look properly at secondary end points such as cardiovascular disease and mortality.

Recently the Losartan Intervention for End-point Reduction in Hypertension (LIFE) trial compared losartan with a beta blocker (atenolol) in patients with left ventricular hypertrophy.[145] The primary composite end point of cardiovascular mortality, fatal/non-fatal stroke, and fatal/non-fatal myocardial infarction was reduced by 14.6% (p<0.009) in the losartan compared with atenolol group, despite similar blood pressures (Figure 59, p69). Benefit was particularly noted with a 26% reduction in stroke.

Reported evidence for cardiovascular benefit with angiotensin II receptor antagonists also comes from human studies suggesting reduction/normalization of structural alterations in small resistance arteries and some studies, but not all, showing regression of left ventricular hypertrophy.[146] Further studies in heart failure are awaited.

In conclusion, angiotensin II receptor antagonists can now be considered as suitable first-line agents for managing hypertension in diabetes, particularly because of their excellent metabolic and side-effect profiles and evidence for renal (and perhaps cardiovascular) protection. These agents may be particularly useful also in the elderly because of their excellent tolerability, once daily dosing and their particular benefit on systolic hypertension.

> *It is clear that drugs from all antihypertensive classes may be needed to reach target levels*

The need for combination therapy

Although renin-angiotensin system inhibitors should normally be first-line treatment for hypertension in diabetes, it is clear that drugs from all antihypertensive classes may be needed to reach target levels. Choice of drug will depend on a range of issues, including patient preference, efficacy and tolerability. It is worrying that only a small percentage of hypertensive patients generally reach the new recommended targets. Indeed, the recent Health Survey for England suggested only 6% of hypertensive patients were reaching the British Hypertension Society guideline blood pressure target of less than 140/85mmHg (Figure 60).[147]

> *Only 6% of hypertensive patients were reaching the British Hypertension Society guideline blood pressure target of less than 140/85mmHg*

Several studies have clearly shown in diabetic patients that combining drugs from different antihypertensive classes will normally be necessary to reach target levels. It is equally clear that in the UK and elsewhere there is a massive amount of undertreatment.

It is also important to realize the evidence base for cardiac and renal protection with renin-angiotensin system inhibitors is with higher doses, and such doses should normally be used for maintenance

	Blood pressure ≥160/95mmHg	Blood pressure ≥140/90mmHg
Population prevalence	20%	40%
Proportion aware of their blood pressure measurement	60%	40%
Proportion on treatment	50%	26%
Proportion controlled	27%	6%

Of those on treatment, 60% were on one drug; 6% on two or more drugs

Fig. 60. Figures from the Health Survey for England[147] **highlighting low rates of hypertension treatment and target achievement.**

after titration in diabetic patients. There is also the interesting finding that combining ACE inhibitors and angiotensin II receptor antagonists produces an additive effect in lowering blood pressure, so this is another combination treatment option.[148]

Future developments

If we add together all the evidence from the various clinical trials, we can estimate that risk of cardiovascular end points and mortality could be reduced by around 75% if all the evidence was applied systematically and aggressively to all diabetic patients (see Figure 26, p28).[149] This is a salutatory thought because there is clearly much undertreatment of cardiovascular risk factors in diabetic patients.

In the near future we are likely to see new indications for established treatments as well as new therapies for cardiovascular risk/cardiovascular disease in diabetic patients. The fact that statins, for example, reduce inflammatory markers which are surrogates for cardiovascular risk suggests an area that needs further examination.

Other areas being explored include the possibility of reducing cardiovascular risk with glitazones through improving insulin resistance, and using the new rapid-acting insulin secretagogues, which restore early-phase insulin secretion and reduce postprandial hyperglycaemia, in the context of reduction in cardiovascular risk.

It is clear, however, that we already have significant evidence on which to base management strategies. We also have the drugs to do the

❝ Risk of cardiovascular end points and mortality could be reduced by around 75% if all the evidence was applied systematically and aggressively to all diabetic patients ❞

The national service framework for diabetes places emphasis on:

- A primary care led service, but with strong collaborative links with secondary care

- Organisation of care through multidisciplinary and multiprofessional working

- Emphasis on vascular risk reduction through:
  - lifestyle changes
  - aggressive screening for and management of hypertension, dyslipidaemia and glycaemia
  - reduction in amputation rates, blindness and renal failure
  - patient empowerment and a more holistic approach to diabetes management

Fig. 61. Key points from the Government's national service framework for diabetes.

job. The major problem is putting results of trials into clinical practice. One hopes the Government's national service framework for coronary heart disease[32] and its recently published national service framework for diabetes[150] will help (Figure 61).

One approach being developed in Birmingham and Coventry, initially tested in the Asian population with high risk of type 2 diabetes and cardiovascular disease, is to use a culturally sensitive, multiprofessional community-based approach to cardiovascular risk management in type 2 diabetic patients.[151] This involves randomizing practices to "usual" care or to active intervention with Asian link workers, diabetes specialist nurses and extra practice nurse time. All practices are given the same information, including data on glycaemia, lipids and blood pressure.

Already in the active practices after the first year of intervention there has been a significant reduction in cardiovascular risk. It is intended this study, presently in its pilot stage, will be extended to encompass many more patients and practices with robust economic assessment and for a longer period of time. A fundamental part of this study is use of algorithms for management with clear lifestyle and pharmacological pathways to achieve target HbA_{1c}, blood pressure and cholesterol levels. The care pathways are nurse run and so far proving very successful.

In summary, we now have evidence that multiple risk factor intervention can significantly reduce cardiovascular morbidity and mortality in diabetic patients. The real challenge is to put the evidence into practice.

> *One approach being developed is to use a culturally sensitive, multiprofessional community-based approach to cardiovascular risk management in type 2 diabetic patients*

Case study 1

"New registration" patient with type 2 diabetes

History

Mr M is a 51-year-old Caucasian who attends for a registration check with the practice nurse. He has a clerical job with the police force, which he dislikes. He has recently divorced and lives alone. He was diagnosed with diabetes 6 years ago and has been taking gliclazide for 18 months. He is on no other medication. He admits to irregular attendance at the clinic but he has seen his optometrist for retinopathy screening. He has a family history of coronary heart disease (his father and paternal uncle had heart attacks in their 60s), but there is no known history of diabetes. He smokes heavily and drinks 30 units of alcohol per week.

Examination

The practice nurse documents a BMI of 27kg/m^2, blood pressure 156/95mmHg, blood glucose 13.4mmol/l mid-morning, and glucose+++, protein+ on urinalysis. He books a 10-minute appointment with his GP the same morning to 'set up a repeat prescription' for gliclazide. He has problems getting time off work for medical appointments.

" Good communication is a cornerstone of these first consultations "

Targets for Mr M's treatment

- **Blood pressure** <140/80mmHg
- **Total cholesterol** <5mmol/l
- **LDL cholesterol** <3mmol/l
- **HbA$_{1c}$** <7mmol/l

Management issues

Engaging Mr M through good communication is a cornerstone of these first consultations and will nurture compliance with the lifestyle measures and life-long drug therapy that will be necessary. He is a high risk for cardio-vascular disease and from the preliminary history alone the need for more medication is clear. A detailed history and full examination, including an ECG is needed to exclude established cardiovascular disease.

Hypertension Three readings above the target of 140/90mmHg will con-firm the diagnosis of hypertension and the need for treatment with either an ACE inhibitor or an angiotensin II receptor antagonist. Urea, electrolytes and creatinine should be tested with his baseline blood tests, and these will

Achieving Mr M's management targets

1. Lifestyle changes
- **Smoking**
- **Alcohol consumption**
- **Exercise and diet.**

2. Pharmacotherapy
- **ACE inhibitor or angiotensin II receptor antagonist (to reduce blood pressure and protect the heart and kidneys)**
- **Almost certainly another antihypertensive(s) in combination**
- **Statin**
- **Aspirin (75mg once daily)**
- **Metformin plus possibly another oral antidiabetic agent**

" Adequate explanation of the concepts of coronary heart disease risk will help compliance "

need to be repeated 2 weeks after starting treatment. Appointment times for checking response to treatment should be as convenient as possible to aid compliance and provide opportunities for continued education.

Glycaemic control With a BMI of 27kg/m² Mr M is overweight. His HbA_{1c} is likely to be high and this should be explained clearly. Once home blood glucose monitoring is established (Figure 62) and dietary education has taken place a switch to metformin would be appropriate. There is a small but significant risk of lactic acidosis with metformin and excess alcohol. Hopefully, he will follow the advice to reduce his alcohol intake considerably. An HbA_{1c} of less than 7% is the target.

Lipids It is almost certain that the coronary heart disease risk calculation will be more than 15% and that Mr M will need to start on a statin. Adequate explanation of the concepts of coronary heart disease risk will help compliance. Side-effects can sometimes be a problem but it is worth trying a few alternatives if necessary.

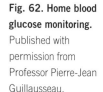

Fig. 62. Home blood glucose monitoring.
Published with permission from Professor Pierre-Jean Guillausseau.

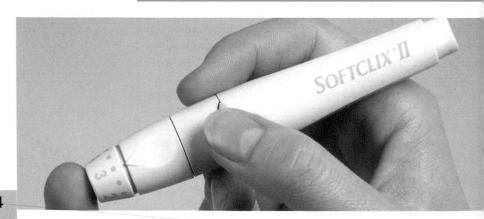

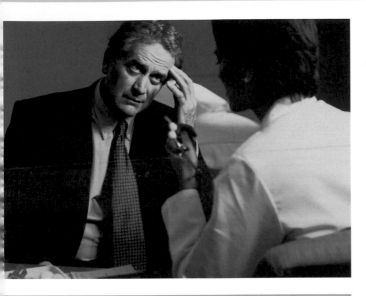

Fig. 63. Education needs to be accessible, continuing and meaningful.

Aspirin Because Mr M is diabetic and hypertensive, the risk of coronary heart disease will be reduced further by 75mg aspirin daily.

Proteinuria The presence of proteinuria on urinalysis is very significant as a predictive marker of cardiovascular disease outcomes and mortality and the development of overt nephropathy. Mr M should be asked to submit an overnight urine collection for albumin excretion rate or albumin/creatinine ratio. A renal ultrasound is necessary to rule out a renal cause for the proteinuria. Controlling his hypertension is critical to management.

Smoking His recent divorce and dislike of his job provide ongoing stresses, which feed Mr M's smoking habit. He will need support and involvement in a smoking cessation programme to tackle this major contributor to his high coronary heart disease risk.

Lifestyle Making an impact on our patients' lifestyle is undoubtedly the most challenging part of management. Mr M's coronary heart disease risk will reduce considerably if he stops smoking, loses weight, eats healthily, drinks less alcohol and exercises. Helping to improve patients' self-esteem and general motivation is a more effective approach than too much directive and authoritarian "medical advice".

Education This needs to be accessible, continuing and meaningful for Mr M (Figure 63). Much can take place away from the clinic or surgery, for example through membership of Diabetes UK, relevant web sites and so on (see Appendix 3).

Regular surveillance This will ensure early diagnosis of Mr M's inevitable cardiovascular disease, which will improve outcomes considerably.

❝ Making an impact on our patients' lifestyle is undoubtedly the most challenging part of management ❞

| Case study 2 |
| Poorly controlled diabetes |

History

Mrs W is a 47-year-old Afro-Caribbean who has had type 2 diabetes for 14 years. She works in the medical records department of the hospital. She is a non-smoker. She has a strong family history of diabetes and stroke. Her diabetes care has been inconsistent and she tends to present at times of crisis. Her hospital and primary care case notes are a testament to her "lost to follow up" status at many clinics. Her last hospital attendance was at the eye clinic 6 months ago when she had focal laser treatment for left eye maculopathy.

She now presents to the A&E department because her left foot has become swollen, red and painful over the previous 24 hours (Figures 64 and 65). She is admitted, and unfortunately her left foot infection becomes gangrenous necessitating amputation of her second and third toes. While in hospital, she continues on the basal bolus regime of insulin established 2 years previously. Her blood sugar control is very uneven, but she ascribes this to her dislike of hospital food and her poor post-operative appetite. Her blood pressure is elevated on a few occasions and the need for this to be checked as an outpatient is highlighted.

Two weeks later she is seen for follow up at the diabetic clinic. She presents as a well-dressed, cheerful and intelligent woman at ease with her diabetes. Her foot feels comfortable and is healing. Arrangements are made for her to see the orthotist. She reports that her blood sugar profiles have settled somewhat since her discharge but her readings are often erratic "just as they usually are".

On taking a history, it becomes clear Mrs W has a limited understanding of the principles of her insulin regime and the dietary requirements of diabetes. She has a reactive approach to insulin doses and food intake.

66On taking a history, it becomes clear Mrs W has a limited understanding of the principles of her insulin regime and the dietary requirements of diabetes 99

Examination

On clinical examination her blood pressure is 148/94mmHg. Cardiovascular examination is normal. She has evidence of severe peripheral neuropathy and on dilated fundoscopy has progression of her retinopathy (Figure 66).

Investigation results show an HbA_{1c} of 11.7% (similar to documented results over the previous 3 years), cholesterol 7.2mmol/l, HDL cholesterol 3.4mmol/l, fasting triglycerides 4.6mmol/l, and a 10-year coronary heart disease risk of 13%. Her creatinine is marginally elevated and U&Es, thyroid function and liver function tests are normal. Urinalysis during her in-patient stay consistently showed proteinuria, and her albumin excretion rate on 24-hour urine collection is over 300mg/24hr.

Management issues

Macrovascular disease Despite her 10-year coronary heart disease risk, Mrs W carries a high risk for macrovascular disease. She has raised blood pressure, raised fasting triglycerides, probable established diabetic nephropathy and poorly controlled diabetes. She has a family history of stroke. To reduce this risk, the aims of immediate treatment are as follows.

•*Control blood pressure.* The target for Mrs W's blood pressure is 125/75mmHg. This is particularly important given her probable nephropathy. She should be started on an ACE inhibitor or an

"Despite her 10-year coronary heart disease risk, Mrs W carries a high risk for macrovascular disease"

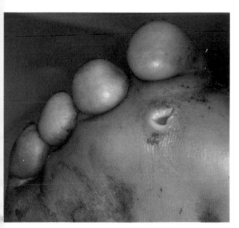
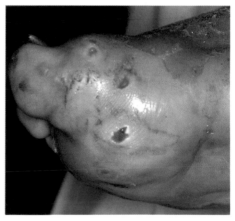

Figs. 64 and 65. Foot lesions in a patient with neglected type 2 diabetes. The multiple fistulae indicate diffusion of the abscess to the whole forefoot. Published with permission from Professor Pierre-Jean Guillausseau.

angiotensin II receptor antagonist, initially in a small dose (eg ramipril 1.25mg or irbesartan 150mg) with titration of dose against response. Her renal function should be monitored 2 weeks after starting the drug and repeated after each increase in dose.

A second agent may be needed, for example bendrofuazide 2.5mg daily or indapamide MR 1.25mg daily. Lifestyle measures, such as exercise, low-salt diet, are important and should always be emphasized.

•*Reduce lipids.* Mrs W should be started on a statin, for example

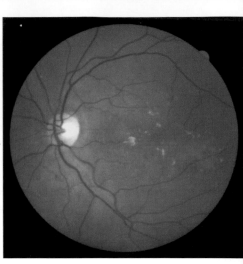

Fig. 66. Diabetic maculopathy. The numerous hard exudates scattered over the macula region indicate high risk for involvement of the fovea and loss of central vision. Published with permission from Professor Roy Taylor.

"Regular HbA$_{1c}$ measurements, which will hopefully show an improvement, will reinforce the impact of Mrs W's efforts "

atorvastatin 40mg once daily. The target is to get her fasting triglycerides below 2.3mmol/l and cholesterol below 5mmol/l. Liver function tests should be checked 1 to 3 months after starting and then annually.

•*Aspirin.* Mrs W should be started on aspirin 75mg unless there are contraindications.

Microvascular complications Mrs W has established progressive microvascular complications of diabetes. The following can significantly reduce the progression of these complications.

•*Education.* Mrs W has had type 2 diabetes for a long time but seems indifferent to the consequences of poor control. She may have underlying long-term problems in accepting her diabetes and living with the daily burden of monitoring, healthy eating and so on. She may have difficulties understanding the concepts being explained to her, despite her apparent confidence. A comprehensive education programme needs to be organized to ensure she gains as full an understanding as possible of her problems.

•*Improve diabetes control.* Mrs W is on a basal bolus regime of insulin. Her control is very poor. The reasons for this will only be apparent if she can be established on regular home blood glucose monitoring, and the results looked at in conjunction with a detailed diary of food/activity/symptoms and so on. She needs a review with the dietitian and diabetes specialist nurse. She may need her insulin regime changed after this. Sensitivity to emerging difficulties is essential. Regular HbA$_{1c}$ measurements, which will hopefully show an improvement, will reinforce the impact of Mrs W's efforts.

•*Regular review.* Mrs W has defaulted from appointments and doesn't appear to have engaged with the diabetes team in either primary or secondary care. She will need accessible support on a day-to-day basis. The diabetes specialist nurse and practice nurse are of paramount importance and can communicate any continuing concerns about diabetes control, physical and mental well being to other members of the team. Establishing a trusting relationship with Mrs W will improve compliance with appointments and treatment.

•*Regular follow up.* Mrs W needs tertiary care for her diabetes complications. This will inevitably mean more appointments and with her track record for non-attendance, there will be a concern about how compliant she will be. Good communication as well as sensitivity to difficulties with 'time off from work' and so on will help her gain confidence in the care system. Hopefully, once her complications have stabilized somewhat she can be followed up mainly at the general diabetes clinic with intercurrent primary care review.

•*Medication compliance.* Controlling hypertension with an ACE inhibitor or angiotensin II receptor antagonist will help slow the progression of her nephropathy and will help her retinopathy. Regular blood tests for lipids, renal function, and liver function should be carried out.

•Using a diabetes co-operation card is essential with a patient like Mrs W whose care pathway is complicated and whose disease is progressive. She should feel the professionals are all aware of each other's role allowing her to feel more at ease with her considerable problems.

66Sensitivity to emerging difficulties is essential99

Management targets for Mrs W

1. Reduce of risk of macrovascular disease
- **Control blood pressure – target 125/75mmHg**
- **Reduce lipids – cholesterol <5mmol/l; triglycerides <2.3mmol/l**
- **Aspirin 75mg once daily**
- **Dietary measures – low salt diet**
- **Exercise**

2. Slow progression of microvascular complications
- **Education programme**
- **Improve diabetes control – target HbA$_{1c}$ <7%**
- **Regular diabetes specialist nurse /practice nurse review**
- **Regular eye clinic /foot clinic /renal clinic review until stabilized**
- **Encourage compliance with medication**

3. Communication
- **Diabetes co-operation card**

66 Using a diabetes co-operation card is essential with a patient like this 99

Case study 3

"Cardiabetes"

History

Mr B is a 60-year-old of South Asian origin whose type 2 diabetes was diagnosed 5 years ago. His past history illustrates how the informal term "cardiabetes" perfectly describes the large group of people moving between cardiology and diabetes out-patients who are also the "frequent consulters" in primary care. He was first diagnosed with hypertension at age 39. This was treated in primary care and his blood pressure readings were 130-150/90mmHg on treatment. His BMI was 27kg/m^2. He had his first myocardial infarct at age 44 and had two further infarcts before his triple artery bypass graft at age 47. He was fairly well with good exercise tolerance until age 53. He then found his job as a factory foreman too much and retired on medical grounds.

His diabetes came to light when he was 55. The diagnosis was made on a glucose tolerance test when his GP found glycosuria but a normal random blood sugar. He had no diabetes symptoms, but Mr S wasn't too surprised as many of his of relatives were diabetic. He was initially treated with metformin (echocardiogram had shown good ventricular function), but insulin was added 18 months ago because of poor diabetes control. He is now on twice daily insulin injections using a fixed mixture (40 units twice daily), metformin, nicorandil, frusemide, bisoprolol, lisinopril, simvastatin, amlodipine isosorbide mononitrate and aspirin. His BMI is 32kg/m^2, blood pressure 140/80mmHg, HbA$_{1c}$ is 11%, but his cholesterol is 4mmol/l, triglycerides are 2.0mmol/l, and renal function tests are normal. He has no proteinuria.

Insulin has not improved his overall diabetes control and his obesity and low levels of activity are worsening his obvious insulin resistance. He has recently experienced chest pain on exertion and has had to undergo a coronary angiogram. His non-grafted coronary artery and one of the grafted arteries have stenozed. Improving his diabetes control is essential to improve outcome for any surgical interventions. However, his cardiac prognosis is guarded.

Management issues

Diabetes control An HbA$_{1c}$ of 11% is unacceptably high and poor diabetes control must be a major factor in Mr B's lack of well-being. Lethargy secondary to hyperglycaemia prevents him from exercising even the limited amount that his cardiac reserve allows. He needs a

"Poor diabetes control must be a major factor in Mr B's lack of well-being"

"Lethargy secondary to hyperglycaemia prevents him from exercising even the limited amount that his cardiac reserve allows."

detailed assessment from the dietitian with the aim of weight reduction followed by a review with the diabetes specialist nurse. He would benefit from a change in insulin regime. A basal bolus regime, using the new long-acting insulin glargine (providing a more even level of basal insulin throughout 24 hours) with a fast-acting soluble insulin injection before each meal is worth a trial. He should continue with metformin and the dose of this could be increased up to 1g twice daily unless he develops heart failure.

Blood pressure and lipids Mr B's blood pressure needs to remain below 125/75mmHg. His lipids are satisfactory, but should be monitored every 6 months, as increases in the dose of simvastatin may be necessary.

Renal function Mr B should have renal function tests every 6 months. Fortunately there is no proteinuria and with continued good control of his hypertension, the risk of nephropathy is reduced.

Liaison with cardiologists Mr B's coronary heart disease has progressed since his bypass and he may now face further intervention. Liaison, particularly concerning diabetes control will ensure the best possible outcome.

Psychological problems Mr B's heart disease and diabetes have dramatically altered Mr B's life. His enforced retirement at a young age will have affected his self-esteem and feeling of worth. His life is punctuated by hospital visits and he seems to be "getting worse not better". He is vulnerable to becoming clinically depressed and this will exacerbate the difficulties in achieving good diabetes control. The diabetes team and the GP/practice nurse need to be aware of this and arrange counselling and start antidepressants if indicated.

Mr B's case also illustrates the need for screening for diabetes in those at risk. It is likely he was diabetic for some time before diagnosis, given his early development of coronary heart disease and his family history.

He is vulnerable to becoming clinically depressed and this will exacerbate the difficulties in achieving good diabetes control

Management targets for Mr B

- Weight reduction
- Improve diabetes control
- Close review of blood pressure and lipids
- Monitor renal function
- Liaise with cardiologists
- Awareness of psychological issues

81

Case study 4
Impaired glucose tolerance

History

Mrs N is a 42-year-old Caucasian who is married with four children. She works as a classroom assistant and is also involved in caring for her ageing parents. She comes from a large family where there is a history of hypertension and coronary heart disease in male siblings. She has a sister with polycystic ovaries who has had difficulty conceiving. She has two maternal uncles with a history of type 2 diabetes diagnosed in their 70s. All the family are "big" and Mrs N has "struggled with her weight" since she was a teenager. She is a non-smoker. She presents to the surgery complaining of being "tired all the time" and asking if she can be prescribed something to help her to lose weight.

"Mrs N represents one of the 17% of the UK population who have impaired glucose tolerance"

Examination

On examination she is overweight with a BMI of 34kg/m². Her blood pressure is 145/95mmHg. She appears pale and admits to recent menorrhagia. Clinical examination is otherwise normal. She returns for fasting blood tests and the results are as follows:
- Fasting glucose: 6.5mmol/l
- Cholesterol: 7.4mmol/l
- HDL cholesterol: 1.4mmol/l
- Triglycerides: 2.6 mmol/l
- 10-year coronary heart disease risk: 11.2%
- T4: 14.2mmol/l
- TSH: 1.00mU/l
- LFTs, U&E, creatinine: normal
- Hb: 10.6g/dl, 28% hypochromic.

   A subsequent oral glucose tolerance test showed that Mrs N had impaired glucose tolerance with a fasting glucose of 6.6mmol/l and a 2-hour glucose of 10mmol/l.

Management issues

Impaired glucose tolerance Mrs N represents one of the 17% of the UK population who have impaired glucose tolerance, which must be diagnosed on an oral glucose tolerance test. She carries a high risk of progression to type 2 diabetes. There is increasing evidence for the value of intervention to slow or prevent her progression to frank diabetes. The most striking comes from the Finnish Diabetes Prevention study which targeted over 500 patients with impaired glucose tolerance with a mean age of 55 years and a BMI of 31kg/m2.[152] The intervention group was given lifestyle advice on healthy eating and increased exercise. After 4 years there was a 58% reduction in developing diabetes in the intervention group. Mrs N should therefore be offered detailed dietary and lifestyle advice and be empowered to see how her long-term well-being and risk of morbidity will be affected by prevention of diabetes. Teaching her home blood glucose monitoring is a useful tool to keep her in touch with these concepts. In my experience patients like Mrs N are not keen on this because of cost and inconvenience. She will need repeat fasting blood sugars performed at the surgery annually or earlier if she develops symptoms.

"Impaired glucose tolerance in itself carries an increased risk of cardiovascular disease"

Cardiovascular morbidity and mortality risk Impaired glucose tolerance in itself carries an increased risk of cardiovascular disease. In the Whitehall study,[153] after 20 years of follow up, there was an age-adjusted hazard ratio of coronary heart disease mortality of 2.14 compared with normal controls. The Da Qing study[154] showed a 10-fold increase in the prevalence of ECG abnormalities in Chinese patients with impaired glucose tolerance, compared with normal controls. The DECODE study group last year published data from 13 prospective trials involving over 25,000 participants across Europe. This confirmed that a raised post-challenge glucose level was an independent risk factor for premature death.[155,156]

Close attention therefore needs to be paid to Mrs N's co-existing risk factors of borderline hypertension and raised total cholesterol. Losing weight, reducing the fat and salt content of the diet and increasing exercise have been shown to reduce blood pressure and lipids.

"In my experience patients like Mrs N are not keen on home blood glucose monitoring because of cost and inconvenience"

Anaemia Mrs N has a busy lifestyle and her tiredness is to a large extent explained by her anaemia. Correcting this will give her the energy to tackle her general fitness level and increase her motivation to lose weight. She may need further gynaecological investigation, for example to exclude fibroids.

Management targets for Mrs N

- Diet/ weight loss
- Monitoring of blood sugar/annual fasting blood sugar
- Blood pressure checks
- Annual lipids check
- On-going education/lifestyle advice
- Exercise programme

Cardiovascular complications

History

Mrs C is a 63-year-old Caucasian who comes from a family with a strong history of coronary heart disease. She has four siblings who had heart attacks in their 40s. She is a smoker who stops smoking for 3 to 4 months every few years. She has been overweight since the birth of her children. She is a diligent attender at all her appointments. She developed anginal symptoms aged 48 and was referred to the cardiologist. An exercise test confirmed her angina. She became hypertensive a year later. She was found to have glycosuria at around this time and subsequent blood tests confirmed she had developed diabetes.

The focus of care 10 years ago was control of her anginal symptoms, achieving "single figure" blood sugar readings and "reasonable" blood pressure control. Her diabetes required oral hypoglycaemics 6 months after diagnosis and she was taking metformin and gliclazide in addition to diltiazem and isosorbide mononitrate.

She was admitted to the local hospital with an infero-lateral myocardial infarction 10 years ago when she was just 54. She made an uncomplicated recovery. She was converted to insulin during her in-patient stay and was started on aspirin. Although hypercholesterolaemia was documented as a diagnosis in her hospital discharge letter, she was not started on a statin but was encouraged to have a low-fat diet. She was eventually started on simvastatin 18 months after her myocardial infarction and ultimately had a good response to this, with cholesterol readings averaging 4.5mmol/l. She had a coronary angiogram 6 months after her myocardial infarction. She was found to have single vessel disease with a blocked right coronary artery (Figure 67) and mildly impaired left ventricular contractility.

Medication

Mrs C's diabetes has been looked after on a shared-care basis. Not surprisingly, the relatively large insulin doses she needed produced weight gain. Her HbA_{1c} readings deteriorated after an initial improvement in the first year after insulin was started. Addition of acarbose, however, produced a significant result in lowering blood sugars and helped reduce insulin dose. Unfortunately, she developed unacceptable side-effects with acarbose and asked for it to be stopped. This was replaced with metformin.

"Not surprisingly, the relatively large insulin doses she needed produced weight gain"

Her medication therefore comprised:
- Humulin M3 twice daily
- Metformin 850mg twice daily
- Aspirin 75mg once daily
- Simvastatin 10mg once daily
- Frusemide 80mg once daily
- Isosorbide mononitrate 60mg once daily
- Ramipril 5mg once daily.

Eleven years after being diagnosed with type 2 diabetes, Mrs C's BMI was 34kg/m², HbA_{1c} 10.6%, cholesterol 4.7mmol/l, and renal, hepatic and thyroid function were normal. An echocardiogram was requested around this time because she complained of increasing dyspnoea and possible orthopnoea. This was essentially normal with good valve and left ventricular function. She was diagnosed with asthma and started on inhalers.

Complications

Six months later, Mrs C was admitted to another hospital as an emergency. She had presented with increasing breathlessness and a productive cough. She spent two weeks as an inpatient and the discharge letter documented type 1 respiratory failure and heart failure. She had impaired renal function on her in-patient blood tests. Her metformin was stopped, but otherwise medication was unchanged. She recovered well and now reports that her breathlessness is "back to the way it always is".

However, she has hyperglycaemic symptoms. Her current blood tests show an HbA_{1c} of 11.7%, cholesterol of 3.9mmol/l and normal renal, hepatic and thyroid function. Her BMI is 37kg/m² and she continues to smoke. Her blood pressure is 130/75mmHg.

Management issues

Mrs C presents a real challenge, but her history illustrates the cardiac nature of diabetes and the difficulty achieving risk and morbidity reduction in some patients. Her family history is a "non-modifiable" risk factor, but alerts one to the high risk. Her smoking raises the risk significantly and she has shown a willingness and discipline to stop, albeit sporadically. It would be worth offering her ongoing smoking cessation advice and support and prescribing, say, nicotine patches. Her probable chronic obstructive pulmonary disease makes this very important and improved lung function is a tangible reward for her efforts here.

"Her history illustrates the cardiac nature of diabetes and the difficulty there is achieving risk and morbidity reduction in some patients"

85

Her diabetes control is poor and this must be affecting her well-being considerably. Now that her renal function is known to have returned to normal, she could be prescribed metformin again. However, there is a possibility she has significant heart failure and this would be a contraindication to prescribing metformin . She therefore warrants another echocardiogram.

Her insulin regime should be altered. She would benefit from a change to insulin glargine, the new long-acting insulin analogue, which would provide even background basal insulin levels. Depending on the response to this, varying doses of a short-acting insulin analogue could be added before meals. She has a high degree of insulin resistance, which makes high doses of insulin necessary whatever the regime adopted.

Patients like Mrs C can understandably feel a sense of hopelessness and passivity about their diabetes and the complications they have developed. Attending multiple clinics and seeing different doctors, nurses and so on can be dispiriting. Much of her day-to-day care can take place in the surgery and the practice nurse, supported by the diabetes specialist nurse, can help Mrs C gain confidence about changing insulin doses.

Thiazide diuretics

Drug	Trade name	Preparation	Strength	Doses used in hypertension (adult)	Comments	Side-effects
Bendroflumethiazide (bendrofluazide)	Neo-NaClex	Tablet	2.5mg, 5mg	25mg mane	Contraindicated in patients with gout; caution in hepatic and renal impairment, pregnancy and breast feeding; higher doses may aggravate diabetes mellitus	Postural hypotension, mild gastrointestinal effects, impotence, hypokalaemia, hypomagnesaemia, hyponatraemia, hypocalcaemia, hypochloraemic alkalosis, hyperuricaemia, gout, hyperglycaemia, altered plasma lipid concentrations
Chlortalidone (chlorthalidone)	Hygroton	Tablet	50mg	25mg mane increasing to 50mg prn	Contraindicated in patients with gout; caution in hepatic and renal impairment, pregnancy and breast feeding; higher doses may aggravate diabetes mellitus	Postural hypotension, mild gastrointestinal effects, impotence, hypokalaemia, hypomagnesaemia, hyponatraemia, hypocalcaemia, hypochloraemic alkalosis, hyperuricaemia, gout, hyperglycaemia, altered plasma lipid concentrations
Cyclopenthiazide	Navidrex	Tablet	500mcg	25mg mane increasing to 500mcg prn	Drug of choice for elderly patients contraindicated in patients with gout; use with other drugs if hypertension is not controlled with low dose; higher doses may aggravate diabetes mellitus	Postural hypotension, mild gastrointestinal effects, impotence, hypokalaemia, hypomagnesaemia, hyponatraemia, hypocalcaemia, hypochloraemic alkalosis, hyperuricaemia, gout, hyperglycaemia, altered plasma lipid concentrations
Indapamide	Natrilix, Natrilix SR	Tablet, M/R tablet	2.5mg, 1.5mg	2.5mg mane, 1.5mg mane swallowed whole	Contraindicated in patients with gout; caution in hepatic and renal impairment, pregnancy and breast feeding; may aggravate diabetes mellitus less than other thiazides	Hypokalaemia, headache, dizziness, fatigue, muscle cramps, nausea, anorexia, diarrhoea, constipation, rashes
Metolazone	Metenix 5	Tablet	5mg	5mg mane; maintenance 5mg on alternate days	Drug of choice for elderly patients; contraindicated in patients with gout; caution in hepatic and renal impairment, pregnancy and breast feeding; higher doses may aggravate diabetes mellitus	Postural hypotension, mild gastrointestinal effects, impotence, hypokalaemia, hypomagnesaemia, hyponatraemia, hypocalcaemia, hypochloraemic alkalosis, hyperuricaemia, gout, hyperglycaemia, altered plasma lipid concentrations
Xipamide	Diurexan	Tablet	20mg	20mg mane	Drug of choice for elderly patients; contraindicated in patients with gout; caution in hepatic and renal impairment, pregnancy and breast feeding; higher doses may aggravate diabetes mellitus	Gastrointestinal effects, mild dizziness, hypokalaemia and other electrolyte disturbances

Beta adrenoceptor blocking drugs

Drug	Trade name	Preparation	Strength	Doses used in hypertension (adult)	Comments	Side-effects
Acebutolol	Sectral	Capsule	100mg, 200mg	400mg/d increasing to 400mg 2 times/d prn	Contraindicated in asthma, chronic obstructive pulmonary disease and heart block; caution in renal and hepatic impairment, pregnancy and breast feeding	Bradycardia (less likely), heart failure, conduction disorders, bronchospasm, peripheral vasoconstriction (less likely), gastrointestinal effects, fatigue, sleep disturbance
		Tablet	400mg			
Atenolol	Tenormin 25	Tablet	25mg	50mg/d	Contraindicated in asthma, chronic obstructive pulmonary disease and heart block; accumulates in renal impairment (reduce dose); caution in hepatic impairment, pregnancy and breast feeding	Bradycardia, heart failure, conduction disorders, bronchospasm, peripheral vasoconstriction, gastrointestinal effects, fatigue, sleep disturbance (less likely)
	Tenormin LS	Tablet	50mg			
	Tenormin	Tablet	100mg			
Betaxolol	Kerlone	Tablet	20mg	20-40mg/d (elderly 10mg/d)	Contraindicated in asthma, chronic obstructive pulmonary disease and heart block; relatively cardioselective; accumulates in renal impairment (reduce dose); caution in hepatic impairment, pregnancy and breast feeding	Bradycardia, heart failure, conduction disorders, bronchospasm, peripheral vasoconstriction, gastrointestinal effects, fatigue, sleep disturbance
Bisoprolol	Cardicor	Tablet	1.25mg, 2.5mg, 3.75mg, 5mg, 7.5mg, 10mg	5-10mg/d (max 20mg/d)	Contraindicated in asthma, chronic obstructive pulmonary disease and heart block; relatively cardioselective; accumulates in hepatic and renal impairment (reduce dose); caution in pregnancy and breast feeding	Bradycardia, heart failure, conduction disorders, bronchospasm, peripheral vasoconstriction, gastrointestinal effects, fatigue, sleep disturbance
	Emcor	Tablet	5mg, 10mg	5-10mg/d (max 20mg/d)		
	Monocor	Tablet	5mg, 10mg			
Carvedilol	Eucardic	Tablet	3.125mg, 6.25mg, 12.5mg, 25mg	12.5-25mg/d (elderly 12.5mg/d) (max 50mg/d)	Contraindicated in asthma, chronic obstructive pulmonary disease, heart block and hepatic impairment; caution in renal impairment, pregnancy and breast feeding	Postural hypotension, dizziness, headache, fatigue, gastrointestinal effects, bradycardia

Beta adrenoceptor blocking drugs

Drug	Trade name	Preparation	Strength	Doses used in hypertension (adult)	Comments	Side-effects
Celiprolol	Celectol	Tablet	200mg 400mg	200mg mane increasing to 400mg prn	Contraindicated in asthma, chronic obstructive pulmonary disease and heart block; accumulates in renal impairment (reduce dose); caution in hepatic impairment, pregnancy and breast feeding; take before food	Headache, dizziness, fatigue, nausea, somnolence
Labetolol	Trandate	Tablet	100mg, 200mg, 400mg	100-200mg 2 times/d (elderly 50mg 2 times/d initially) (max 2.4g/d)	Contraindicated in asthma, chronic obstructive pulmonary disease, heart block and hepatic impairment; caution in renal impairment, pregnancy and breast feeding take with or after food	Postural hypotension, tiredness, weakness, headache, rashes, scalp tingling, difficulty in micturition, epigastric pain, nausea, vomiting, liver damage
Metoprolol	Betaloc	Tablet	50mg, 100mg	100mg/d; maintenance 100-200mg/d	Contraindicated in asthma, chronic obstructive pulmonary disease, heart block; accumulates in hepatic impairment (reduce dose); caution in hepatic impairment, pregnancy and breast feeding; M/R formulations should be swallowed whole	Bradycardia, heart failure, conduction disorders, bronchospasm, peripheral vasoconstriction, gastrointestinal effects, fatigue, sleep disturbance
	Betaloc-SA	M/R tablet	200mg			
	Lopressor	Tablet	50mg, 100mg,			
	Lopressor SR	M/R tablet	200mg			
Nadolol	Corgard	Tablet	40mg, 80mg	80mg/d (max 240mg/d)	Contraindicated in asthma, chronic obstructive pulmonary disease and heart block; caution in renal and hepatic impairment, pregnancy and breast feeding	Bradycardia, heart failure, conduction disorders, bronchospasm, peripheral vasoconstriction, gastrointestinal effects, fatigue, sleep disturbance (less likely)
Nebivolol	Nelibet	Tablet	5mg	5mg/d (2.5mg/d initially elderly)	Contraindicated in asthma, chronic obstructive pulmonary disease, heart block and hepatic impairment; accumulates in renal impairment (reduce dose); caution in pregnancy and breast feeding	Bradycardia, heart failure, conduction disorders, bronchospasm, peripheral vasoconstriction, gastrointestinal effects, fatigue, sleep disturbance, oedema, headache, depression, visual disturbances, impotence

Beta adrenoceptor blocking drugs

Drug	Trade name	Preparation	Strength	Doses used in hypertension (adult)	Comments	Side-effects
Oxprenolol	Trasicor	Tablet	20mg, 40mg, 80mg	80–160mg/d in 2–3 divided doses (max 320mg)	Contraindicated in asthma, chronic obstructive pulmonary disease and heart block; caution in renal and hepatic impairment, pregnancy and breast feeding; M/R formulation should be swallowed whole	Bradycardia (less likely), heart failure, conduction disorders, bronchospasm, peripheral vasoconstriction (less likely), gastrointestinal effects, fatigue, sleep disturbance
	Slow-Trasicor	M/R tablet	160mg	160mg/d (max 320mg/d)		
Pindolol	Visken	Tablet	5mg, 15mg	5mg 2–3 times/d increasing to 15–30mg/d (max 45mg/d)	Contraindicated in asthma, chronic obstructive pulmonary disease, heart block; accumulates in renal impairment (reduce dose); caution in hepatic impairment, pregnancy and breast feeding	Bradycardia, heart failure, conduction disorders, bronchospasm, peripheral vasoconstriction, gastrointestinal effects, fatigue, sleep disturbance
Propranolol	Inderal	Tablet	10mg, 40mg, 80mg	80mg 2 times/d; maintenance 160–320mg/d	Contraindicated in asthma, chronic obstructive pulmonary disease and heart block; caution in renal and hepatic impairment, pregnancy and breast feeding; M/R formulations should be swallowed whole	Bradycardia, heart failure, conduction disorders, bronchospasm, peripheral vasoconstriction, gastrointestinal effects, fatigue, sleep disturbance
	Half-Inderal LA	M/R capsule	80mg	80–160mg/d		
	Inderal LA	M/R capsule	160mg	160–320mg/d		
Timolol	Betim	Tablet	10mg	10mg/d (max 60mg/d in divided doses if above 20mg)	Contraindicated in asthma, chronic obstructive pulmonary disease and heart block; caution in renal and hepatic impairment, pregnancy and breast feeding	Bradycardia, heart failure, conduction disorders, bronchospasm, peripheral vasoconstriction, gastrointestinal effects, fatigue, sleep disturbance

Alpha adrenoceptor blocking drugs

Drug	Trade name	Preparation	Strength	Doses used in hypertension (adult)	Comments	Side-effects
Doxazosin	Cardura	Tablet	1mg, 2mg	1mg/day initially, increasing to 2mg and 4mg/d	Contraindicated in urinary incontinence; caution in hepatic impairment; M/R formulations should be swallowed whole	Postural hypotension, dizziness, vertigo, headache, fatigue, asthenia, oedema, somnolence, nausea, rhinitis
	Cardura XL	M/R tablet	4mg, 8mg	8mg pm (max 16mg/d)		
Indoramin	Baratol	Tablet	25mg	25mg 2 times/d initially (max 300mg) in 2-3 divided doses)	Contraindicated in urinary incontinence and established heart failure; caution in hepatic and renal impairment	Sedation, dizziness, depression, failure of ejaculation, dry mouth, nasal congestion, extrapyramidal effects, weight gain
Prazosin	Hypovase	Tablet	500mcg, 1mg, 2mg, 5mg	500mcg 2-3 times/d initially (max 20mg/d)	Contraindicated in urinary incontinence and congested heart failure; reduce dose in hepatic and renal impairment; caution in pregnancy and breast feeding	Postural hypotension, drowsiness, weakness, dizziness, headache, lack of energy, nausea, palpitations, urinary frequency, incontinence, priapism
Terazosin	Hytrin	Tablet	1mg, 2mg, 5mg, 10mg	1mg nocte increasing to 2-10mg/d (max 20mg)	Contraindicated in urinary incontinence	Postural hypotension, dizziness, lack of energy, peripheral oedema, urinary frequency, priapism

Angiotensin converting enzyme inhibitors

Drug	Trade name	Preparation	Strength	Doses used in hypertension (adult)	Comments	Side-effects
Captopril	Capoten	Tablet	12.5mg, 25mg, 50mg	12.5mg 2 times daily (6.25mg 2 times daily) increasing to 25mg 2 times daily with diuretic, elderly (max 150mg)	Contraindicated in renovascular disease, aortic stenosis, outflow tract obstruction, porphyria and pregnancy; caution in renal impairment	Renal impairment, persistent dry cough, angioedema, rash, pancreatitis, upper respiratory tract effects, gastrointestinal effects, liver function abnormalities, headache, dizziness, fatigue, malaise, taste disturbance, myalgia, arthralgia, tachycardia, serum sickness, weight loss, stomatitis, photosensitivity, flushing
Cilazapril	Vascace	Tablet	500mcg, 1mg, 2.5mg, 5mg	1mg/d (500mcg/d with diuretic, renal impairment, elderly), maintenance 1-2.5mg/d (max 5mg/d)	Contraindicated in renovascular disease, aortic stenosis, outflow tract obstruction, severe hepatic impairment and pregnancy; caution in renal impairment	Renal impairment, persistent dry cough, angioedema, rash, pancreatitis, upper respiratory tract effects, gastrointestinal effects, liver function abnormalities, headache, dizziness, fatigue, malaise, taste disturbance, myalgia, arthralgia, dyspnoea, bronchitis

Angiotensin converting enzyme inhibitors

Drug	Trade name	Preparation	Strength	Doses used in hypertension (adult)	Comments	Side-effects
Enalapril	Innovace	Tablet	2.5mg, 5mg, 10mg, 20mg	5mg/d (2.5mg/d with diuretic, renal impairment, elderly), maintenance 20mg/d (max 40mg/d)	Contraindicated in renovascular disease, aortic stenosis, outflow tract obstruction, porphyria and pregnancy; caution in renal and hepatic impairment	Renal impairment, persistent dry cough, angioedema, rash, pancreatitis, upper respiratory tract effects, gastrointestinal effects, liver function abnormalities, headache, dizziness, fatigue, malaise, taste disturbance, myalgia, arthralgia, palpitations, arrhythmias, chest pain, syncope, cerebrovascular accident, anorexia, stomatitis, dermatological effects, confusion, depression, nervousness, insomnia, impotence
Fosinopril	Staril	Tablet	10mg, 20mg	10mg/d (less with diuretic), maintenance 10-40mg/d (max 40mg/d)	Contraindicated in renovascular disease, aortic stenosis, outflow tract obstruction, severe hepatic impairment, porphyria and pregnancy; caution in renal impairment	Renal impairment, persistent dry cough, angioedema, rash, pancreatitis, upper respiratory tract effects, gastrointestinal effects, liver function abnormalities, headache, dizziness, fatigue, malaise, taste disturbance, myalgia, arthralgia, chest pain, musculoskeletal pain
Imidapril	Tanatil	Tablet	5mg, 10mg, 20mg	5mg/d (2.5mg/d with diuretic, heart failure, cerebrovascular disease, angina, renal or hepatic impairment, elderly), maintenance 10mg/d (max 20mg/d)	Contraindicated in renovascular disease, aortic stenosis, outflow tract obstruction and pregnancy; caution in renal and hepatic impairment	Renal impairment, persistent dry cough, angioedema, rash, pancreatitis, upper respiratory tract effects, gastrointestinal effects, liver function abnormalities, headache, dizziness, fatigue, malaise, taste disturbance, myalgia, arthralgia, dry mouth, glossitis, abdominal pain, bronchitis, sleep disturbances, depression, confusion, blurred vision, tinnitus, impotence
Lisinopril	Carace	Tablet	2.5mg, 5mg, 10mg, 20mg	2.5mg/d, maintenance 10-20mg/d (max 40mg/d)	Contraindicated in renovascular disease, aortic stenosis, outflow tract obstruction and pregnancy; caution in renal impairment	Renal impairment, persistent dry cough, angioedema, rash, pancreatitis, upper respiratory tract effects, gastrointestinal effects, liver function abnormalities, headache, dizziness, fatigue, malaise, taste disturbance, myalgia, tachycardia, cerebrovascular accident, myocardial infarction, dry mouth, confusion, mood changes, asthenia, sweating, impotence
	Zestril		2.5mg, 5mg, 10mg, 20mg			

Angiotensin converting enzyme inhibitors

Drug	Trade name	Preparation	Strength	Doses used in hypertension (adult)	Comments	Side-effects
Moexipril	Perdix	Tablet	7.5mg, 15mg	7.5mgd (3.75mgd with diuretic, renal or hepatic impairment, elderly), maintenance 15-30mg/d (max 30mg/d)	Contraindicated in renovascular disease, aortic stenosis, outflow tract obstruction and pregnancy; caution in renal and hepatic impairment	Renal impairment, persistent dry cough, angioedema, rash, pancreatitis, upper respiratory tract effects, gastrointestinal effects, liver function abnormalities, headache, dizziness, fatigue, malaise, taste disturbance, myalgia, tachycardia, arrhythmias, angina, chest pain, syncope, cerebrovascular accident, myocardial infarction, appetite and weight changes, dry mouth, photosensitivity, flushing, nervousness, mood changes, anxiety, drowsiness sleep disturbance
Perindopril	Coversyl	Tablet	2mg, 4mg	2mg/d (less with diuretic), maintenance 4mg/d (max 8mg/d)	Contraindicated in renovascular disease, aortic stenosis, outflow tract obstruction and pregnancy; caution in renal and hepatic impairment	Renal impairment, persistent dry cough, angioedema, rash, pancreatitis, upper respiratory tract effects, gastrointestinal effects, liver function abnormalities, headache, dizziness, fatigue, malaise, taste disturbance, myalgia, tachycardia, asthenia, flushing, mood and sleep disturbances
Quinapril	Accupro	Tablet	5mg, 10mg, 20mg, 40mg	10mg/d (2.5mg with diuretic, renal impairment, elderly), maintenance 20-40mg/d (max 80mg/d)	Contraindicated in renovascular disease, aortic stenosis, outflow tract obstruction and pregnancy; caution in renal and hepatic impairment	Renal impairment, persistent dry cough, angioedema, rash, pancreatitis, upper respiratory tract effects, gastrointestinal effects, liver function abnormalities, headache, dizziness, fatigue, malaise, taste disturbance, myalgia, tachycardia, asthenia, chest pain, oedema, flatulence, nervousness, insomnia, blurred vision, impotence, back pain, myalgia
Ramipril	Tritace	Tablet	1.25mg, 2.5mg, 5mg, 10mg	1.25mg/d (less with diuretic), maintenance 2.5-5mg/d (max 10mg/d)	Contraindicated in renovascular disease, aortic stenosis, outflow tract obstruction and pregnancy; caution in renal and hepatic impairment	Renal impairment, persistent dry cough, angioedema, rash, pancreatitis, upper respiratory tract effects, gastrointestinal effects, liver function abnormalities, headache, dizziness, fatigue, malaise, taste disturbance, myalgia, tachycardia, arrhythmias, angina, chest pain, myocardial infarction, loss of appetite, dry mouth, dermatological effects, confusion, nervousness, depression, anxiety, impotence, bronchitis, muscle cramps

Angiotensin converting enzyme inhibitors

Drug	Trade name	Preparation	Strength	Doses used in hypertension (adult)	Comments	Side-effects
Trandolapril	Gopten	Capsule	500mcg, 1mg, 2mg	500mcg/d (less with diuretic), maintenance 1–2mg/d (max 4mg/d)	Contraindicated in renovascular disease, aortic stenosis, outflow tract obstruction, and pregnancy; caution in renal and hepatic impairment	Renal impairment, persistent dry cough, angioedema, rash, pancreatitis, upper respiratory tract effects, gastrointestinal effects, liver function abnormalities, headache, dizziness, fatigue, malaise, taste disturbance, myalgia, tachycardia, arrhythmias, angina, chest pain, cerebral haemorrhage, myocardial infarction, dry mouth, dermatological effects, asthenia, alopecia, dyspnoea, bronchitis
	Odrik	Capsule	500mcg, 1mg, 2mg			

Angiotensin II receptor antagonists

Drug	Trade name	Preparation	Strength	Doses used in hypertension (adult)	Comments	Side-effects
Candesartan	Amias	Tablet	2mg, 4mg, 8mg, 16mg	4mg/d (2mg in hepatic and renal impairment), maintenance 8mg (max 16mg)	Contraindicated in pregnancy and breast feeding; caution in aortic or mitral valve stenosis, obstructive hypertrophic cardiomyopathy, renal and hepatic impairment	Symptomatic hypotension, hyperkalaemia, upper respiratory tract symptoms, abdominal pain, back pain, arthralgia, myalgia, nausea, headache, dizziness, peripheral oedema, rash
Eprosartan	Teveten	Tablet	300mg, 400mg, 600mg	600mg/d (300mg/d >75 years, hepatic and renal impairment), maintenance 800mg/d	Contraindicated in pregnancy and breast feeding; caution in aortic or mitral valve stenosis, obstructive hypertrophic cardiomyopathy, renal and hepatic impairment	Symptomatic hypotension, hyperkalaemia, flatulence, dizziness, arthralgia, rhinitis, hypertriglyceridaemia
Irbesartan	Aprovel	Tablet	75mg, 150mg, 300mg	150mg/d (75mg/d >75 years), maintenance 300mg/d	Contraindicated in pregnancy and breast feeding; caution in aortic or mitral valve stenosis, obstructive hypertrophic cardiomyopathy, renal and hepatic impairment	Symptomatic hypotension, hyperkalaemia, diarrhoea, dyspepsia, flushing, tachycardia, dizziness, asthenia, myalgia, rash, urticaria
Losartan	Cozzar	Tablet	25mg, 50mg, 100mg	50mg/d (25mg/d >75 years, severe renal impairment) (max 100mg/d)	Contraindicated in pregnancy and breast feeding; caution in aortic or mitral valve stenosis, obstructive hypertrophic cardiomyopathy, renal and hepatic impairment	Symptomatic hypotension, hyperkalaemia, diarrhoea, dizziness, taste disturbance, cough, myalgia, migraine, urticaria, pruritus, rash

Angiotensin II receptor antagonists

Drug	Trade name	Preparation	Strength	Doses used in hypertension (adult)	Comments	Side-effects
Telmisartan	Micardis	Tablet	20mg, 40mg, 80mg	40mg/d (max 80mg/d)	Contraindicated in biliary obstruction, gastric or duodenal ulceration, pregnancy and breast feeding; caution in aortic or mitral valve stenosis, obstructive hypertrophic cardiomyopathy, renal and hepatic impairment	Symptomatic hypotension, hyperkalaemia, gastrointestinal effects, pharyngitis, back pain, myalgia
Valsartan	Diovan	Capsule	40mg, 80mg, 160mg	80mg/d (40mg/d >75 years, renal and hepatic impairment) (max 160mg/d)	Contraindicated in biliary obstruction, cirrhosis, pregnancy and breast feeding; caution in aortic or mitral valve stenosis, obstructive hypertrophic cardiomyopathy, renal and hepatic impairment	Symptomatic hypotension, hyperkalaemia, fatigue

Calcium channel blockers

Drug	Trade name	Preparation	Strength	Doses used in hypertension (adult)	Comments	Side-effects
Amlodipine	Istin	Tablet	5mg, 10mg	5mg/d (max 10mg/d)	Contraindicated in cardiogenic shock, unstable angina, aortic stenosis, pregnancy and breast feeding; caution in renal and hepatic impairment	Headache, oedema, fatigue, nausea, flushing, dizziness, gum hyperplasia, rashes
Felodipine	Plendil	Tablet	2.5mg, 5mg, 10mg	5mg mane (2.5mg mane elderly), maintenance 5-10mg mane (max 20mg mane) swallowed whole	Contraindicated in unstable angina, uncontrolled heart failure, aortic stenosis, within 1 month of myocardial infarction and pregnancy; caution in renal and hepatic impairment	Flushing, headache, palpitations, dizziness, fatigue, gravitational oedema
Isradipine	Prescal	Tablet	2.5mg	2.5mg 2 times/d (25mg 2 times/d elderly, hepatic or renal impairment), maintenance 2.5-10mg/d (max 10mg 2 times/d)	Contraindicated in tight aortic stenosis, sick sinus syndrome and pregnancy; caution in renal and hepatic impairment	Headache, flushing, dizziness, tachycardia, palpitations, localised peripheral oedema

Calcium channel blockers

Drug	Trade name	Preparation	Strength	Doses used in hypertension (adult)	Comments	Side-effects
Lacidipine	Motens	Tablet	2mg, 4mg	2mg mane, maintenance 4mg mane (max 6mg mane)	Contraindicated in aortic stenosis, within 1 month of myocardial infarction, pregnancy and breast feeding; caution in renal and hepatic impairment	Headache, flushing, oedema, dizziness, palpitations
Lercanidipine	Zanidip	Tablet	10mg	10mg/d (max 20mg/d) before food	Contraindicated in aortic stenosis, unstable angina, uncontrolled heart failure, within 1 month of myocardial infarction and pregnancy; caution in renal and hepatic impairment, left ventricular dysfunction, sick sinus syndrome	Flushing, peripheral oedema, palpitations, tachycardia, headache, dizziness, asthenia
Nicardipine	Cardene	Capsule	10mg, 20mg	20mg 3 times/d, maintenance 60-120mg/d	Contraindicated in cardiogenic shock, aortic stenosis, unstable angina, within 1 month of myocardial infarction, pregnancy and breast feeding; caution in congestive heart failure, impaired left ventricular function, renal and hepatic impairment	Dizziness, headache, peripheral oedema, flushing, palpitations, nausea
	Cardene SR	M/R capsule	30mg, 45mg	30mg 2 times/d, maintenance 30-60mg 2 times/d swallowed whole		
Nifedipine	Adalat LA	M/R tablet	20mg,30 mg, 60mg	40mg 20mg/d initially	Contraindicated in cardiogenic shock, advanced aortic stenosis, unstable angina, within 1 month of myocardial infarction, porphyria; caution in pregnancy and breast feeding, congestive heart failure, impaired left ventricular function, renal and hepatic impairment; patients should be maintained on the same brand because of variations in clinical effect; all formulations should be swallowed whole	Headache, flushing, dizziness, lethargy, tachycardia, palpitations, gravitational oedema, rash, pruritus, urticaria, nausea, constipation, visual disturbances, gum hyperplasia, paraesthesia, impotence, depression
	Adalat Retard	M/R tablet	10mg, 20mg	10mg 2 times/d (max 40mg 2 times/d)		
	Adipine MR	M/R tablet	10mg, 20mg	10mg 2 times/d (max 40mg 2 times/d)		
	Coracten SR	M/R capsule	10mg, 20mg	20mg 2 times/d, maintenance 10-40mg 2 times/d		
	Coracten XL	M/R capsule	30mg, 60mg	30mg/d (max 90mg/d)		
	Fortipine LA 40	M/R tablet	40mg	40mg/d (max 80mg/d)		

Calcium channel blockers

Drug	Trade name	Preparation	Strength	Doses used in hypertension (adult)	Comments	Side-effects
Nisoldipine	Syscor MR	M/R tablet	10mg, 20mg, 30mg	10mg mane (max 40mg mane) swallowed whole	Contraindicated in cardiogenic shock, aortic stenosis, unstable angina, within 1 month of myocardial infarction, hepatic impairment, pregnancy and breast feeding; caution in renal impairment	Gravitational oedema, headache, flushing, tachycardia, palpitations, dizziness, asthenia, gastrointestinal effects

Fibrates

Drug	Trade name	Preparation	Strength	Doses used in lipid regulation (adult)	Comments	Side-effects
Bezafibrate	Bezalip	Tablet	200mg	200mg 3 times/d after food	May reduce the risk of coronary heart disease in patients with low HDL cholesterol or with raised triglycerides. Contraindicated in severe hepatic impairment, hyperalbuminaemia, primary biliary cirrhosis, gall bladder disease, nephrotic syndrome, pregnancy and breast feeding; caution in renal impairment (reduce dose)	Gastrointestinal effects (e.g. nausea, anorexia, gastric pain), pruritus, urticaria, impotence, headache, dizziness, vertigo, fatigue, alopecia; myelotoxicity (with myasthenia or myalgia) is a particular risk in patients with renal impairment
	Bezalip Mono	Tablet	400mg	400mg/d after food and swallowed whole		
Ciprofibrate	Modalim	Tablet	100mg	100mg/d	May reduce the risk of coronary heart disease in patients with low HDL cholesterol or with raised triglycerides. Contraindicated in severe hepatic impairment, hyperalbuminaemia, primary biliary cirrhosis, gall bladder disease, nephrotic syndrome, pregnancy and breast feeding; caution in renal impairment (reduce dose)	Gastrointestinal effects (e.g. nausea, anorexia, gastric pain), pruritus, urticaria, impotence, headache, dizziness, vertigo, fatigue, alopecia; myelotoxicity (with myasthenia or myalgia) is a particular risk in patients with renal impairment

Drug	Trade name	Preparation	Strength	Doses used in lipid regulation (adult)	Comments	Side-effects
Fibrates						
Finofibrate	Lipantil Micro 67	Capsule	67mg	3 capsules/d (range 2-4 capsules) after food	May reduce the risk of coronary heart disease in patients with low HDL cholesterol or with raised triglycerides. Contraindicated in severe hepatic and renal impairment, gall bladder disease, pregnancy and breast feeding; caution in renal impairment (reduce dose), monitor hepatic function, photosensitivity to ketoprofen	Gastrointestinal effects (e.g. nausea, anorexia, gastric pain), pruritus, urticaria, impotence, headache, dizziness, vertigo, fatigue, alopecia, rash, photosensitivity, raised serum transaminases, hepatitis; myelotoxicity (with myasthenia or myalgia) is a particular risk in patients with renal impairment
	Lipantil Micro 200	Capsule	200mg	1 capsule/d after food		
	Lipantil Micro 267	Capsule	267mg	1 capsule/d after food		
	Supralip 160	M/R tablet	160mg	1 tablet/d after food and swallowed whole		
Statins						
Atorvastatin	Lipitor	Tablet	10mg, 20mg, 40mg, 80mg	10mg/d	May reduce the risk of coronary heart disease in patients with diabetes mellitus; contraindicated in active hepatic disease, pregnancy and breast feeding; caution in history of hepatic disease, monitor hepatic function	Reversible myositis, headache, alterations in hepatic function tests, gastrointestinal effects (abdominal pain, flatulence, diarrhoea, nausea, vomiting), rash, hypersensitivity reactions (including rash, angioedema, anaphylaxis), insomnia, anorexia, paraesthesia, peripheral neuropathy, alopecia, pruritus, impotence, chest pain, hypoglycaemia, hyperglycaemia
Fluvastatin	Lescol	Capsule	20mg, 40mg	20-40mg in the evening (max 80mg/d)	May reduce the risk of coronary heart disease in patients with diabetes mellitus; contraindicated in active hepatic disease, severe renal impairment, pregnancy and breast feeding; caution in history of hepatic disease, monitor hepatic function	Reversible myositis, headache, alterations in hepatic function tests, gastrointestinal effects (abdominal pain, flatulence, diarrhoea, nausea, vomiting), rash, hypersensitivity reactions (including rash, angioedema, anaphylaxis), insomnia
	Lescol XL	M/R tablet	80mg			
Pravastatin	Lipostat	Tablet	10mg, 20mg, 40mg	10-40mg nocte	May reduce the risk of coronary heart disease in patients with diabetes mellitus; contraindicated in active hepatic disease, pregnancy and breast feeding; caution in history of hepatic disease, monitor hepatic function	Reversible myositis, headache, alterations in hepatic function tests, gastrointestinal effects (abdominal pain, flatulence, diarrhoea, nausea, vomiting), rash, hypersensitivity reactions (including rash, angioedema, anaphylaxis), chest pain, fatigue

Statins

Drug	Trade name	Preparation	Strength	Doses used in lipid regulation (adult)	Comments	Side-effects
Rosuvastatin	Crestor	Tablet	10mg	10mg once daily; before treatment the patient should be placed on a cholesterol-lowering diet to continue curing treatment; dose should be individualised according to the treatment goal and patient response using consensus guidelines; can be increased to 20mg once daily after 4 weeks; an increase of dose to 40mg should only be considered for severe hypercholesterol-aemia with high cardiovascular risk (in particular familial hypercholesterolaemia) if the treatment goal is not achieved on 20mg and there will be routine follow-up	Indicated in primary hypercholesterolaemia (type IIa including heterozygous familial hypercholesterolaemia) or mixed dys-lipidaemia (type IIb) as an adjunct to diet if not responding to diet and other nonpharmacological treatments; indicated for homozygous familial hypercholesterolaemia as an adjunct to diet and other lipid lowering treatment or if such treatments are inappropriate; contraindicated if hypersensitive to rosuvastatin or any excipients, in active liver disease (including unexplained persistent elevations of serum transaminases and any serum transaminase elevation over three times upper limit of normal [ULN]), in severe renal impairment, in myopathy, in any serious acute condition predisposing to renal failure secondary to rhabdomyolysis, in those on ciclosporin (ciclosporin increases rosuvastatin AUC), during pregnancy and breast feeding, in premenopausal women not using contraception; consider assessing renal function in follow-up of those on 40mg; measure creatine kinase (CK) – not following strenuous exer-cise – before treatment – if over five times ULN do not start; liver function tests before and 3 months after start of treatment; caution if predisposing factors for rhabdomyolysis – clinical monitoring recommended; coadministration with gemfibrozil not recommended; caution if coadministered with fibrates or niacin; caution if excessive alcohol or history of liver disease; treat underlying cause of secondary hypercholesterolaemia before treatment; caution with vitamin K antagonists (monitor INR), erythromycin, oral contraception, hormone replacement	Common (>1/100, <1/10) – headache, dizziness, constip-ation, nausea, abdo-minal pain, myalgia, asthenia; rare (>1/10,000, <1/1300) – myopathy – uncomplicated myalgia and myopathy (rarely rhabdomyolysis in patients receiving 80mg) – all improved on cessation of therapy; proteinuria on dipstick testing, in particular with higher doses, especially 40mg; dose-related increase in CK; dose-related increase in transaminases

Statins

Drug	Trade name	Preparation	Strength	Doses used in lipid regulation (adult)	Comments	Side-effects
Simvastatin	Zocor	Tablet	10mg, 20mg, 40mg, 80mg	10mg nocte, range 10–80mg nocte	May reduce the risk of coronary heart disease in patients with diabetes mellitus; contraindicated in active hepatic disease, porphyria, pregnancy and breast feeding; caution in severe renal impairment, history of hepatic disease, monitor hepatic function	Reversible myositis, headache, alterations in hepatic function tests, gastrointestinal effects (abdominal pain, flatulence, diarrhoea, nausea, vomiting), rash, hypersensitivity reactions (including rash, angioedema, anaphylaxis), alopecia, amnesia, dizziness, paraesthesia, peripheral neuropathy, hepatitis, jaundice, pancreatitis

Anti-obesity agents

Drug	Trade name	Preparation	Strength	Doses used in obesity (adult)	Comments	Side-effects
Orlistat	Xenical	Capsule	120mg	120mg up to 3 times daily immediately before, during or up to 1 hour after each main meal	Pancreatic lipase inhibitor which inhibits the absorption of dietary fat used as adjunct to dietary control; contraindicatedin chronic malabsorption syndrome, cholestasis, pregnancy and breast feeding	Liquid oily stools, faecal urgency, flatulence, abdominal and rectal pain, headache, menstrual irregularities, anxiety, fatigue
Sibutramine	Reductil	Capsule	10mg, 15mg	10–15mg mane	Centrally acting appetite suppressant; contraindicated in history of major eating disorders, psychiatric illness, Gilles de la Tourette syndrome, history of coronary artery disease, congestive heart failure, tachycardia, peripheral arterial occlusive disease, arrhythmias, cerebrovascular disease, uncontrolled hypertension, hyperthyroidism, pregnancy and breast feeding; caution in hepatic and renal impairment	Constipation, anorexia, dry mouth, insomnia, nausea, tachycardia, palpitations, hypertension, vasodilatation, paraesthesia, headache, anxiety, sweating, taste disturbance, blurred vision

Sulphonylureas

Drug	Trade name	Preparation	Strength	Doses used to lower blood glucose (adult)	Comments	Side-effects
Glibenclamide	Daonil Semi Daonil Euglycon	Tablet Tablet Tablet	5mg 2.5mg 2.5mg, 5mg	2.5-5mg with or immediately after breakfast	Contraindicated in severe hepatic and renal impairment, porphyria, pregnancy (substitute insulin), breast feeding, elderly (use shorter acting sulphonylurea); caution in mild to moderate hepatic and renal impairment	Gastrointestinal disturbances (nausea, vomiting, diarrhoea, constipation), disturbances in hepatic function (cholestatic jaundice, hepatitis), hypersensitivity reactions (mainly allergic skin reactions shortly after starting therapy)
Gliclazide	Diamicron Diamicron MR	Tablet M/R tablet	80mg 30mg	40-80mg/d (max single dose 160mg, divided dose 320mg/d) 30mg with breakfast (max 120mg/d)	Contraindicated in severe hepatic and renal impairment, porphyria, pregnancy (substitute insulin), breast feeding; caution in mild to moderate hepatic and renal impairment	Gastrointestinal disturbances (nausea, vomiting, diarrhoea, constipation), disturbances in hepatic function (cholestatic jaundice, hepatitis), hypersensitivity reactions (mainly allergic skin reactions shortly after starting therapy)
Glimepiride	Ameryl	Tablet	1mg, 2mg, 3mg, 4mg	1mg/d before or with breakfast, range 1-4mg/d (max 6mg)	Contraindicated in severe hepatic and renal impairment, porphyria, pregnancy (substitute insulin), breast feeding, elderly (use shorter acting sulphonylurea); caution in mild to moderate hepatic and renal impairment	Gastrointestinal disturbances (nausea, vomiting, diarrhoea, constipation), disturbances in hepatic function (cholestatic jaundice, hepatitis), hypersensitivity reactions (mainly allergic skin reactions shortly after starting therapy)
Glipizide	Glibenese Minodiab	Tablet Tablet	5mg 2.5mg	2.5-5mg before breakfast (max single dose 15mg, divided dose 20mg/d)	Contraindicated in severe hepatic and renal impairment, porphyria, pregnancy (substitute insulin), breast feeding, elderly (use shorter acting sulphonylurea); caution in mild to moderate hepatic and renal impairment	Gastrointestinal disturbances (nausea, vomiting, diarrhoea, constipation), disturbances in hepatic function (cholestatic jaundice, hepatitis), hypersensitivity reactions (mainly allergic skin reactions shortly after starting therapy), dizziness, drowsiness
Gliquidone	Glurenorm	Tablet	30mg	15mg before breakfast increasing to 45-60mg/d in 2 or 3 divided doses (max single dose 60mg, divided dose 180mg/d)	Contraindicated in severe hepatic and renal impairment, porphyria, pregnancy (substitute insulin), breast feeding, elderly (use shorter acting sulphonylurea); caution in mild to moderate hepatic and renal impairment	Gastrointestinal disturbances (nausea, vomiting, diarrhoea, constipation), disturbances in hepatic function (cholestatic jaundice, hepatitis), hypersensitivity reactions (mainly allergic skin reactions shortly after starting therapy), headache, tinnitus

Sulphonylureas

Drug	Trade name	Preparation	Strength	Doses used to lower blood glucose (adult)	Comments	Side-effects
Tolbutamide	Generic	Tablet	500mg	0.5–1.5g /d with or immediately after breakfast (max 2g/d in divided doses)	Contraindicated in severe hepatic and renal impairment, porphyria, pregnancy (substitute insulin), breast feeding; caution in mild to moderate hepatic and renal impairment	Gastrointestinal disturbances (nausea, vomiting, diarrhoea, constipation), disturbances in hepatic function (cholestatic jaundice, hepatitis), hypersensitivity reactions (mainly allergic skin reactions shortly after starting therapy)

Biguanides

Drug	Trade name	Preparation	Strength	Doses used to lower blood glucose (adult)	Comments	Side-effects
Metformin	Glucophage	Tablet	500mg, 850mg	500mg before breakfast increasing after 1 week to 500mg before breakfast and evening meal and then 500mg before breakfast, lunch and evening meal prn (usual max 2g/d)	Most suitable drug for obese patients when dieting has failed to control diabetes; contraindicated in hepatic and renal impairment, ketoacidosis, predisposition to lactic acidosis, heart failure, severe infection and trauma, dehydration, alcohol dependence, pregnancy, breast feeding	Gastrointestinal disturbances (anorexia, nausea, vomiting, diarrhoea), abdominal pain, metallic taste, lactic acidosis - rare, withdraw treatment, decreased vitamin B12 absorption

Other antidiabetic agents

Drug	Trade name	Preparation	Strength	Doses used to lower blood glucose (adult)	Comments	Side-effects
Acarbose	Glucobay	Tablet	50mg, 100mg	50mg/d increasing to 50mg 3 times/d then 100mg 3 times daily after 6-8 weeks prn (max 200mg 3 times daily); swallow whole immediately before food	Contraindicated in inflammatory bowel diseases (Crohn's disease, ulcerative colitis), partial intestinal obstruction; hepatic impairment, severe renal impairment, hernia, history of abdominal surgery, pregnancy and breast feeding	Flatulence, soft stools, diarrhoea (tends to decrease with time), abdominal distention and pain, abnormal liver function tests, skin reactions, ileus, oedema, jaundice, hepatitis
Nateglinide	Starlix	Tablet	60mg, 120mg, 180mg	60mg 3 times/d before main meals (max 180mg 3 times daily)	Use in combination with metformin; contraindicated in diabetic ketoacidosis, severe hepatic impairment, pregnancy and breast feeding; caution in debilitated and malnourished patients, moderate hepatic impairment, substitute insulin during intercurrent illness and surgery	Hypoglycaemia, hypersensitivity reactions (pruritus, rashes, urticaria)

Other antidiabetic agents

Drug	Trade name	Preparation	Strength	Doses used to lower blood glucose (adult)	Comments	Side-effects
Pioglitazone	Actos	Tablet	15mg, 30mg	15–30mg/d	Used in combination with metformin or a sulphonylurea but not with insulin (risk of heart failure); contraindicated in hepatic impairment, history of heart failure, pregnancy and breast feeding; monitor liver function during treatment	Gastrointestinal disturbances, weight gain, oedema, anaemia, headache, visual disturbances, dizziness, arthralgia, haematuria, impotence, hypoglycaemia, fatigue, sweating, altered blood lipids, proteinuria
Repaglinide	NovoNorm	Tablet	500mcg, 1mg, 2mg	500mcg/d before main meals (max single dose 4mg, max 16mg/d in divided doses)	Contraindicated in diabetic ketoacidosis, severe hepatic impairment, pregnancy and breast feeding; caution in debilitated and malnourished patients, renal impairment, substitute insulin during intercurrent illness and surgery	Abdominal pain, diarrhoea, constipation, nausea, vomiting, hypoglycaemia, hypersensitivity reactions (prorates, rashes, urticaria)
Rosiglitazone	Avandia	Tablet	4mg, 8mg	4mg/d increasing to 8mg/d (in combination with metformin) after 8 weeks prn	Used in combination with metformin or a sulphonylurea but not with insulin (risk of heart failure); contraindicated in hepatic impairment, history of heart failure, pregnancy and breast feeding; monitor liver function during treatment	Gastrointestinal disturbances, headache, anaemia, fatigue, weight gain, oedema, hypoglycaemia, dizziness, drowsiness, paraesthesia, rash, alopecia, dyspnoea, altered blood lipids, thrombocytopenia, pulmonary oedema

Cholesterol absorption inhibitor

Drug	Trade name	Preparation	Strength	Doses used in lipid regulation (adult)	Comments	Side-effects
Ezetimibe	Ezetrol	Tablet	10mg	10mg once daily. If patient is also being treated with a bile acid sequestrant, give Ezetrol at least 2 hours before or 4 hours after the bile acid sequestrant	Indicated in primary hypercholesterolaemia coadministered with a statin as adjunctive therapy to diet in patients who are not appropriately controlled with a statin alone or as adjunctive therapy to diet in patients for whom a statin is considered to be inappropriate or is not tolerated; also indicated in homozygous familial hypercholesterolaemia coadministered with a statin as adjunctive therapy to diet and in homozygous sitosterolaemia as adjunctive therapy to diet; contraindicated if any hypersensitivity to the active substance or any of the excipients; when coadministered with a statin, contraindicated during pregnancy and breast feeding, in active liver disease, if there are unexplained persistent elevations in serum transaminases; contraindicated during breast feeding; not recommended in moderate or severe hepatic insufficiency; when coadministered with a statin, carry out liver function tests before starting therapy and thereafter as recommended for the statin; coadministration with fibrates not recommended because safety and efficacy have not been established; caution with ciclosporin – mean AUC for total ezetimibe increases	When used alone: headache, abdominal pain, diarrhoea When coadministered with a statin: headache, fatigue, abdominal pain, constipation, diarrhoea, flatulence, nausea, myalgia, elevation in serum transaminase

Abbreviations

Molecules

ACE	Angiotensin converting enzyme
ATP	Adenosine triphosphate
Hb	Haemaglobin
HbA_{1c}	Glycosylated haemoglobin
HDL	High-density lipoprotein
HMG-CoA	Hydroxy methyl glutaryl coenzyme A
IGF-1	Insulin-like growth factor-1
LDL	Low-density lipoprotein
Na^+	Sodium ion
PAI-1	Plasminogen activator inhibitor type 1
PPARα	Peroxisome proliferator activated receptor alpha
PPARγ	Peroxisome proliferator activated receptor gamma
TG	Triglycerides
VLDL	Very-low-density lipoprotein

Trials

ALLHAT	Antihypertensive and Lipid Lowering to prevent Heart Attack Trial
CAPPP	Captopril Prevention Project
DCCT	Diabetes Control and Complications Trial
DECODE	Diabetes Epidemiology: Collaborative Analysis of Diagnostic Criteria in Europe
HOPE	Heart Outcomes Prevention Evaluation
HOT	Hypertension Optimal Treatment
IDNT	Irbesartan in Diabetic Nephropathy Trial
IRMA-2	Irbesartan in Type 2 Diabetes with Microalbuminuria Study
LIFE	Losartan Intervention for Endpoint Reduction in Hypertension
PROGRESS	Perindopril Protection Against Recurrent Stroke Study
RENAAL	Reduction of Endpoints in NIDDM with the Angiotensin II Antagonist Losartan
SHEP	Systolic Hypertension in the Elderly Programme
SYST-EUR	Systolic Hypertension in Europe
UKPDS	UK Prospective Diabetes Study
XENDOS	Xenical (orlistat) and Prevention of Diabetes in Obese Subjects

Other

BMI	Body mass index
CHD	Coronary heart disease
ECG	Electrocardiogram

HOMA	Homeostasis model assessment
IGT	Imparied glucose tolerance
LFTs	Liver function tests
LVH	Left ventricular hypertophy
MI	Myocardial infarction
RR	Relative risk
RRR	Relative risk reduction
SNS	Sympathetic nervous system
T4	Thyroxine
TSH	Thyroid stimulating hormone
WHO	World Health Organization

Contact information for useful organizations

For the health professional

American College of Cardiology
Heart House, 9111 Old Georgetown Road,
Bethesda, MD 20814-1699, USA
Tel: (800) 253 4636, ext. 694
Fax: (301) 897 9745
Website: http://www.acc.org/

American Diabetes Association
(Attn: National Call Center), 1701 North Beauregard Street,
Alexandria, VA 22311, USA
Tel: (800) 342 2383
Website: http://www.diabetes.org

American Society of Hypertension
148 Madison Avenue, New York,
NY 10016, USA
Tel: 212 696 9099
Fax: 212 696 0711
E-mail: ash@ash-us.org
Website: http://www.ash-us.org/

American Stroke Association
National Center, 7272 Greenville Avenue,
Dallas, TX 75231, USA
Tel: 1 800 242 8721
Website: http://www.strokeassociation.org

Blood Pressure Association
60 Cranmer Terrace, London
SW17 0QS, UK
Tel: 020 8772 4994
Fax: 020 8772 4999
Website: http://www.bpassoc.org.uk

British Cardiac Society
9 Fitzroy Square, London W1T 5HW, UK
Tel: 020 7383 3887
Fax: 020 7388 0903
Website: http://www.bcs.com

107

British Hypertension Society
Blood Pressure Unit, Department of Physiological Medicine, St George's
Hospital Medical School, Cranmer Terrace, London SW17 ORE, UK
Tel: 020 8725 3412
Fax: 020 8725 2959
E-mail: bhsis@sghms.ac.uk
Website: http://www.hyp.ac.uk/bhs

Diabetes Network International
Tel: 020 7828 1516
E-mail: info@dni.org.uk
Website: http://www.dni.org.uk/Ny_DNI_site/frameset.html

Diabetes UK
10 Parkway, London NW1 7AA, UK
Tel: 020 7424 1000
Fax: 020 7424 1001
E-mail: info@diabetes.org.uk
Website: http://www.diabetes.org.uk/home.htm

European Atherosclerosis Society
Secretary, Dr. Sebastiano Calandra, Sezione di Patologia Generale,
Dipartimento di Scienze Biomediche, Universita di Modena e Reggio Emilia,
 Via Campi 287, I-41100 Modena, Italy
Tel: +39 059 2055 423
Fax: +39 059 2055 426
Website://www.elsevier.com/inca/homepage/sab/eas/menu.htm

European Society of Cardiology
The European Heart House, 2035 Route des Colles
B.P. 179 – Les Templiers, FR-06903 Sophia Antipolis, France
Tel: +33 4 92 94 76 00
Fax: +33 4 92 94 76 01
E-mail: webmaster@escardio.org
Website: http://www.escardio.org

European Society of Hypertension
Institute of Clinical Experimental Medicine, Dept of Preventive Cardiology,
Videnska 1958/9. 140 21 Prague 4. Czech Republic
Tel: +1 613 761 4785
Fax: +1 613 761 5309
E-mail: info@eshonline.org
Website: http://www.eshonline.org

For the patient

American Diabetes Association
(see above)

British Heart Foundation
14 Fitzhardinge Street, London W1II 6DH, UK
Tel: 020 7935 0185
Fax: 020 7486 5820
E-mail: internet@bhf.org.uk
Website: http://www.bhf.org.uk

Diabetes Insight
C/o Trefoil Solutions Ltd, 15 Ravenhill Avenue,
Knowle, Bristol, BS3 5DU
Tel: 0117 908 1432
Fax: 0117 908 1433
Website: http://www.diabetes-insight.info/

Diabetes Monitor
5689 Chancery Place, Hamilton, Ohio 45011, USA
E-mail: info@diabetesmonitor.com
Website: http://www.diabetesmonitor.com

Diabetes UK
(see above)

Heart UK
7 North Rd, Maidenhead, Berkshire, SL6 1PE
Tel: 01628 628 638
Fax: 01628 628 698
E-mail: ask@heartukorg.uk
Website: http://www.heartuk.org.uk/

References

1   Zimmet PZ, McCarty DJ, de Courten MP. The global epidemiology of non-insulin-dependent diabetes mellitus and the metabolic syndrome. J Diabetes Complicat 1997;11:60-8.

2   British Diabetic Association. Diabetes in the UK 1996. London: British Diabetic Association, 1995.

3   World Health Organization (Europe) and International Diabetes Federation (Europe). Diabetes care and research in Europe: the St Vincent declaration. Diabet Med 1990;7:360-70.

4   Currie CJ, Kraus D, Morgan CL et al. NHS acute sector expenditure for diabetes: the present, future and excess inpatient cost of care. Diabet Med 1997;14:686-92.

5   Baxter H, Bottomley J, Burns E et al. CODE-2 UK: the annual direct costs of care for people with type 2 diabetes in the UK. Diabet Med 2000;17 (Suppl 1):13.

6   Fisher M, Shaw KM. Diabetes – a state of premature cardiovascular death. Pract Diab Int 2001;18:183-4.

7   Stamler J, Vaccaro O, Neaton JD et al. Diabetes, other risk factors and 12-year mortality for men as screened in the multiple risk factor intervention trial. Diabetes Care 1993;16(2):434-44.

8   Kannel WB, McGee DL. Diabetes and cardiovascular risk factors: the Framingham study. Circulation 1979;59(1):8-13.

9   Panzram G. Mortality and survival in type II (non-insulin-dependent) diabetes mellitus. Diabetologia 1987;30:123-31.

10 Haffner SM, Lehto S, Ronnemaa T et al. Mortality from coronary heart disease in subjects with type 2 diabetes and in non-diabetic subjects with and without prior myocardial infarction. N Engl J Med 1998;339:229-34.

11 Pan WH, Cedres LB, Liu K et al. Relationship of clinical diabetes and asymptomatic hyperglycemia to risk of coronary heart disease mortality in men and women. Am J Epidemiol 1986;123:504-16.

12 Aronson D, Rayfield EJ, Chesebro JH. Mechanisms determining course and outcome of diabetic patients who have had acute myocardial infarction. Ann Intern Med 1997;126:296-306.

13 Singer DE, Moulton AW, Nathan DM. Diabetic myocardial infarction. Interaction of diabetes with other preinfarction risk factors. Diabetes 1989;38:350-7.

14 Tzagournis M. Interaction of diabetes with hypertension and lipids – patients at high risk. An overview. Am J Med 1989;86:50-4.

15 Reaven GM. Role of insulin resistance in human disease: Banting Lecture. Diabetes 1988;37:1595-607.

16 Kuczmarski RJ, Flegal KM, Campbell SM et al. Increasing prevalence of overweight among US adults. The National Health and Nutrition Examination Surveys. 1960 to 1991. J Am Med Ass 1994;272:205-11.

17 Surveys OoPCa. Health Survey for England. London: HMSO, 1991.

18 Bain SC. The effects of diabetes on lipoprotein metabolism. In Dodson PM, Barnett AH (eds). Lipids, Diabetes and Vascular Disease. Second edition. London: Science Press, 1998;15-23.

19 Rowe JW, Young JB, Minaker KL et al. Effect of insulin and glucose infusions on sympathetic nervous system activity in normal man. Diabetes 1981;30:219-25.

20 DeFronzo RA. The effect of insulin on renal sodium metabolism. A review with clinical implications. Diabetologia 1981;21:165-71.

21 Calle EE, Thun MJ, Petrelli JM et al. Body-mass index and mortality in a prospective cohort of US adults. N Engl J Med 1999;341:1097-105.

22 WHO. The Asia-Pacific perspective: redefining obesity and its treatment. Geneva: WHO, 2000.

23 British Nutrition Foundation. Obesity Report of the British Nutrition Foundation Taskforce. Oxford: Blackwell Scientific Ltd, 1999.

24 Lapidus L, Bengtsson C, Larsson B et al. Distribution of adipose tissue and risk of cardiovascular disease and death: a 12 year follow up of participants in the population study of women in Gothenburg, Sweden. Br Med J (Clin Res Ed) 1984;289:1257-61.

25 Larsson B, Svardsudd K, Welin L et al. Abdominal adipose tissue distribution, obesity, and risk of cardiovascular disease and death: 13 year follow up of participants in the study of men born in 1913. Br Med J (Clin Res Ed) 1984;288:1401-4.

26 Balarajan R. Ethnic differences in mortality from ischaemic heart disease and cerebrovascular disease in England and Wales. Br Med J 1985;302:560-4.

27 Colditz GA, Willett WC, Rotnitzky A et al. Weight gain as a risk factor for clinical diabetes mellitus in women. Ann Intern Med 1995;122:481-6.

28 Allahabadia A, Kumar S. Diabetes and Obesity: what is the relationship to cardiovascular disease? In Barnett AH (ed). Diabetes Annual. London: Martin Dunitz, 2002 pp15-39.

29 Ramsay L, Williams B, Johnston G et al. Guidelines for management of hypertension: report of the third working party of the British Hypertension Society. J Hum Hypertens 1999;13:569-92.

30 O'Donnell MJ, Chowdhury TA. Hypertension and nephropathy in diabetes. In Barnett AH, Dodson PM (eds). Hypertension and Diabetes (third edition). London: Science Press Ltd, 2000, pp21-31.

31 Bayly GR, Bartlett WA, Davies PH et al. Laboratory-based calculation of coronary heart disease risk in a hospital diabetic clinic. Diabet Med 1999;16:697-701.

32 Department of Health. National Service Framework for Coronary Heart Disease. London: Department of Health, 2000.

33 National Institute for Clinical Excellence. Management of type 2 diabetes – management of blood pressure and blood lipids. Inherited Clinical Guideline H. London, October 2002.

34 Wilding J, Williams G. Diabetes and obesity. In: Kopelman PG (ed). Clinical obesity. Oxford: Blackwell Science; 1998:308-49.

35 Tuomilehto J, Lindstrom J, Eriksson JG et al. Prevention of type 2 diabetes mellitus by lifestyle among subjects with impaired glucose tolerance. N Engl J Med 2001;344:1343-50.

36 Group DPPR. Reduction in the incidence of type 2 diabetes with lifestyle intervention or metformin. N Engl J Med 2002;346:393-403.

37 Lean ME, Powrie JK, Anderson AS et al. Obesity, weight loss and prognosis in type 2 diabetes. Diabet Med 1990;7:228-33.

38 United Kingdom Prospective Diabetes Study (UKPDS) Group. Intensive blood glucose control with sulphonylureas or insulin compared with conventional treatment and risk of complications in patients with type 2 diabetes (UKPDS 33). Lancet 1998;352:837-53.

39 United Kingdom Prospective Diabetes Study Group. Tight blood pressure control and risk of macrovascular and microvascular complications in type 2 diabetes: UKPDS 38. Br Med J 1998;317:703-13.

40 Hansson L, Zanchetti A, Carruthers SG et al. Effect of intensive blood pressure lowering and low-dose aspirin in patients with hypertension: Principal results of the Hypertension Optimal Treatment (HOT) randomised trial. Lancet 1998;351:1755-62.

41 Curb JD, Pressel SL, Cutler et al. Effect of diuretic-based antihypertensive treatment on cardiovascular disease risk in older diabetic patients with isolated systolic hypertension. Systolic Hypertension in the Elderly Program Cooperative Research Group. JAMA 1996;276:1886-92.

42 Tuomilehto J, Rastenyte D, Birkenhager WH et al. Effect of calcium-channel blockade in older subjects with diabetes and systolic hypertension. Systolic Hypertension in Europe Trial Investigators. N Engl J Med 1999;340: 677-84.

43 Hansson L, Lindholm LH, Niskanen L et al. Effect of angiotensin-converting enzyme inhibition compared with conventional therapy on cardiovascular morbidity and mortality in hypertension: the Captopril Prevention Project (CAPPP) randomised trial. Lancet 1999;3543:611-6.

44 Heart Outcomes Prevention Evaluation Study Investigators. Effects of ramipril on cardiovascular and microvascular outcomes in people with diabetes mellitus: results of the HOPE study and MICRO-HOPE sub-study. Lancet 2000;355:253-9.

45 Scandinavian Simvastatin Survival Study Group. Randomised controlled trial of cholesterol lowering in 4444 patients with coronary heart disease: The Scandinavian Simvastatin Survival Study (4S). Lancet 1994;344:1383-9.

46 Shepherd J, Cobbs SM, Ford I et al. Prevention of coronary heart disease with pravastatin in men with hypercholesterolaemia. N Engl J Med 1995;333:1301-7.

47 Sacks FM, Pfeffer MA, Moye LA et al. The effect of pravastatin on coronary events after myocardial infarction in patients with average cholesterol levels. N Engl J Med 1996;335:1001-9.

48 Downs JR, Clearfield M, Weis S et al. Primary prevention of acute coronary events with lovastatin in men and women with average cholesterol levels. Results of AFCAPS/TexCAPS. Jama 1998;279:1615-22.

49 The Long-Term Intervention with Pravastatin in Ischemic Disease (LIPID) Study Group. Prevention of cardiovascular events and death with pravastatin in patients with coronary heart disease and a broad range of initial cholesterol levels. N Engl J Med 1998;339:1349-57.

50 Heart Protection Study Collaborative Group. MRC/BHF Heart Protection study of cholesterol lowering with simvastatin in 20,536 high risk individuals: a randomised placebo-controlled trial. Lancet 2002;360:7-22.

51 Pyorala K, Pedersen TR, Kjekshus J et al. Cholesterol lowering with simvastatin improves prognosis of diabetic patients with coronary heart disease. Diabetes Care 1997;20:614-20.

52 Diabetes UK. Recommendations for the management of diabetes in primary care (second edition). London: Diabetes UK, October 2000.

53 European Diabetes Policy Group. A desktop guide to type 2 diabetes mellitus. Diabet Med 1999;126:716-730.

54 Sjostrom L, Rissanen A, Andersen T et al. Randomised placebo-controlled trial of Orlistat for weight loss and prevention of weight gain in obese patients. Lancet 1998;352:167-73.

55 Hanif MW, Kumar S. Pharmacological management of obesity. Expert Opin Pharmacotherap 2002;3.1711-8.

56 Effect of intensive blood-glucose control with metformin on complications in overweight patients with Type 2 diabetes (UKPDS 34). UK Prospective Diabetes Study (UKPDS) Group. Lancet 1998;352:854-65.

57 Bailey CJ. Antidiabetic drugs. Br J Cardiol 2000;7:350-60.

58 Lebovitz HE. a-glucosidase inhibitors as agents in the treatment of diabetes. Diabetes Rev 1998;6:132-45.

59 Barnett AH. Insulin-sensitizing agents – Thiazolidinediones (Glitazones). Curr Med Res Opin 2002;18:31s-9s.

60 Barman Balfour JA, Plosker GL. Rosiglitazone. Drugs 1999;57:921-30.

61 Matthews DR, Bakst A, Weston WM et al. Rosiglitazone decreases insulin resistance and improves beta-cell function in patients with type 2 diabetes. Abstr. 858. The 35th Annual Meeting of the European Association for the Study of Diabetes. Diabetologia 1999;42(Suppl 1):228.

62 Day C. Thiazolidinediones: a new class of antidiabetic drugs. Diabet Med 1999;16:179-92.

63 Jones NP, Mather R, Owen S et al. Long-term efficacy of rosiglitazone as monotherapy or in combination with metformin. Diabetologia 2000;43(Suppl 1)A192 (Abstr. 736).

64 Raskin P, Dole JE, Rappaport EB. Rosiglitazone improves glycaemic control in poorly controlled insulin-treated type 2 diabetes (T2D). Diabetes 1999;48(Suppl 1):A94.

65 Schneider R, Egan J, Houser V. Combination therapy with pioglitazone and sulphonylurea in patients with type 2 diabetes. Diabetes 1999;48:A106,0458.

66 Wolffenbuttel BH, Gomis R, Squatrito S et al. Addition of low-dose rosiglitazone to sulphonylurea therapy improves glycaemic control in type 2 diabetic patients. Diabet Med 2000;17:40-7.

67 Bakris GL, Dole JF, Porter LA et al. Rosiglitazone improves blood pressure in patients with type 2 diabetes mellitus. Diabetes 2000;49(Suppl 1):Abstr 388.

68 Dogterom P, Jonkman JHG, Vallance SE et al. No effect on erythropoiesis or premature red cell destruction. Diabetes 1999;48(Suppl 1):A98,Abs 0424.

69 Davies MJ. Insulin secretagogues. In Barnett AH (ed). Current Medical Research and Opinion on Diabetes Mellitus. Newbury, UK: Librapharm, 2002;Vol 18 Suppl 1:S22-30.

70 Avignon A, Radauceanu A, Monnier L. Non fasting glucose is a better marker of diabetes control than fasting plasma glucose in type 2 diabetes. Diabetes Care 1997;20:1822-6.

71 DECODE Study Group on behalf of the European Diabetes Epidemiology Study Group. Glucose tolerance and mortality: comparison of WHO and American Diabetes Association diagnostic criteria. Lancet 1999;354:617-21.

72 Ceriello A. The emerging role of post prandial hyperglycaemic spikes in the pathogenesis of diabetic complications. Diabet Med 1998;15:188-93.

73 Efebvre PJ, Scheen AJ. The post prandial state and risk of cardiovascular disease. Diabet Med 1998;15 (Suppl 4):563-8.

74 Van Gaal LF, Van Acker KL, Damsbo P et al. Metabolic effects of repaglinide, a new oral hypoglycaemic agent in therapy of naïve type 2 diabetics. Diabetologia 1995;38(Suppl 1)164.

75 Moses R, Slobodniuk R, Boyages S et al. Effect of repaglinide addition to metformin monotherapy on glycaemic control in patients with type 2 diabetes. Diabetes Care 1999;22:1:119-24.

76 Kristensen JS, Clauson P, Bayer T et al. The frequency of severe hypoglycaemia is reduced with repaglinide treatment compared with sulphonylurea treatment. Eur J Endocrinol 1999;140:Suppl 1:19.

77 Damsbo P, Clauson P, Marbury TC et al. A double-blind randomized comparison of meal-related glycemic control by repaglinide and glyburide in well controlled type 2 diabetic patients. Diabetes Care 1999;22:5:789-94.

78 Landin-Olsson M, Brogard JM, Erikson J et al. The efficacy of repaglinide administered in combination with bedtime NPH-insulin in patients with type 2 diabetes. A randomized, semi-blinded, parallel-group, multi-center trial. Diabetes 1999;48(Suppl 1) A117.

79 Keilson L, Mather S, Walter JH et al. Synergistic effect of nateglinide and meal administration on insulin secretion in patients with type 2 diabetes mellitus. J Clin Endocrinol Metab 2000;85:108:1-6.

80 Hanefeld M, Dickinson S, Bouter KP et al. Rapid and short-acting mealtime insulin secretion with nateglinide controls both prandial and mean glycemaia. Diabetes Care 2000;23:2:202-7.

81 Horton E, Clinkingbeard C, Gatlin M et al. Nateglinide alone and in combination with metformin improves glycaemic control by reducing mealtime glucose levels in type 2 diabetes. Diabetes Care 2000;23:1660-5.

82. Diabetes Control and Complications Trial Group. The Effect of Intensive Treatment of Diabetes on the Development and Progression of Long-Term Complications in Insulin-Dependent Diabetes Mellitus. N Engl J Med 1993; 329(14):977-86

83 Barnett AH, Owens DR. Insulin analogues. Lancet 1997;349·47-51.

84 Kang S, Brange J, Burch A et al. Subcutaneous insulin absorption explained by insulin's physicochemical properties: evidence from absorption studies of soluble human insulin and insulin analogues in humans. Diabetes Care 1991;14:942-8.

85 Heller SR. Insulin analogues. In Barnett AH (ed). Current Medical Research and Opinion – Diabetes Mellitus. Newbury, UK: Librapharm, 2002;Vol 18(Suppl 1):540-7.

86 Fineberg SE, Fineberg S, Anderson JH et al. Does the use of short-acting (LysPro) human insulin in insulin naïve patients augment the insulin immune response or differ between type I and type II patients? Diabetes 1995;44(Suppl 1):23A.

87 Barnett AH. Basal insulin – answers from analogues? In Practical Diabetes International 2002;19:213-6.

88 Lepore M, Pampanelli S, Fanelli CG et al. Pharmacokinetics and pharmacodynamics of subcutaneous injection of long-acting human insulin analog glargine, NPH insulin, and ultralente human insulin and continuous subcutaneous infusion of insulin lispro. Diabetes 2000;49:2142-8.

89 Pieber TP, Eugene-Jolcine E, Derobert E. Efficacy and safety of HOE 901 versus NPH insulin in patients with type 1 diabetes. Diabetes Care 2000;23:157-62.

90 Rosenstock J, Park G, Zimmerman J. Basal insulin glargine (HOE 901) versus NPH insulin in patients with type 1 diabetes on multiple daily insulin regimens. U.S. Insulin Glargine (HOE 901) Type 1 Diabetes Investigator Group. Diabetes Care 2000;23:1137-42.

91 Ratner RE, Hersch IB, Neifing JL et al. Less hypoglycaemia with insulin glargine in intensive insulin therapy for type 1 diabetes. U.S. Study Group of Insulin Glargine in Type 1 Diabetes. Diabetes Care 2001;23:639-43.

92 Raskin P, Klaff L, Bergenstal R et al. A 16-week comparison of the novel insulin analog insulin glargine (HOE 901) and NPH human insulin used with insulin lispro in patients with type 1 diabetes. Diabetes Care 2000;23:1666-71.

93 Yki-Jarvinen H, Dressler A, Ziemen M. Less nocturnal hypoglycaemia and better post-dinner glucose control with bedtime insulin glargine compared with bedtime NPH insulin combination therapy in type 2 diabetes. HOE 901/3002 Study Group. Diabetes Care 2000;23:1130-6.

94 Rosenstock J, Schwartz SL, Clark CM Jr et al. Basal insulin therapy in type 2 diabetes: 28-week comparison of insulin glargine (HOE 901) and NPH insulin. Diabetes Care 2001;24:631-6.

95 Fonseca V, Bell D, Mecca T. Less symptomatic hypoglycaemia with bedtime insulin glargine (Lantus) compared to bedtime NPH insulin in patients with type 2 diabetes [abstract]. Diabetes 2001;50(Suppl 2):112-3.

96 Raskin P, Park G, Zimmerman J. The effect of HOE 901 on glycaemic control in type 2 diabetes [abstract]. Diabetes 1998;47 (Suppl 1):A103.

97 Massi Benedetti M. Results of a 12-month study: insulin glargine (HOE 901) in combination with oral agents [abstract]. 35th Annual Meeting of the European Association for the Study of Diabetes (EASD), Brussels, 1999.

98 Kurtzhals P, Schaffer L, Sorensen A et al. Correlations of receptor binding and metabolic and mitogenic potencies of insulin analogs designed for clinical use. Diabetes 2000;49:999-1005.

99 McKeague K, Goa KL. Insulin glargine. A review of its therapeutic use as a long-acing agent for the management of type 1 and 2 diabetes mellitus. Drugs 2001;61:1599-624.

00 Kurtzhals P, Havelund S, Jonassen Ib et al. Albumin binding and time action of acylated insulins in various species. J Pharm Sci 1996;85:304-8.

01 Markussen J, Havelund S, Kurtzhals P et al. Soluble, fatty acid acylated insulins bind to albumin and show protracted action in pigs. Diabetologia 1996;39:281-8.

02 Whittingham JL, Havelund S, Jonassen Ib. Crystal structure of a prolonged-acting insulin with albumin-binding properties. Biochemistry 1997;36:2826-31.

03 Kurtzhals P, Havelund S, Jonassen IB et al. Albumin binding of insulins acylated with fatty acids: characterization of the ligand-protein interaction and correlation between binding affinity and timing of the insulin effect in vivo. J Biochem 1995;312:725-31.

04 Gänsslen M. Über inhalation von insulin. Klin Wochenschr 1925;4:71.

05 Klonoff DC. Inhaled insulin. Diabetes Technol Ther 1999;1:307-13.

06 Barnett A. Pulmonary insulin delivery in type 1 and type 2 diabetes. Future Prescriber 2001, May/June:18-21.

07 Heise T, Rave K, Bott S et al. Time-action profile on an inhaled insulin preparation in comparison to insulin lispro and regular insulin. Diabetes 2000;49(Suppl 1):A10.

08 Gelfand RA, Schwartz SL, Horton M et al. Pharmacological reproducibility of pre-meal inhaled insulin is comparable to injected insulin in patients with type 2 diabetes. Diabetes 1998;47(Suppl 1):A99.

09 Kipnes M, Otulana B, Okikawa J et al. Pharmacokinetics and pharmacodynamics of pulmonary insulin delivery via the AERx diabetes management system in type 1 diabetics. Diabetologia 2000;43(Suppl 1):A201.

10 Weiss SR, Berger S, Cheng S-L et al. Adjunctive therapy with inhaled insulin type 2 diabetic patients failing oral agents: a multicenter phase II trial. Diabetes 1999;48(Suppl 1):A12.

11 Skyler JS, Cefalu WT, Kourides IA et al on behalf of the Inhaled Insulin Phase II Study Group. Efficacy of inhaled insulin in type 1 diabetes mellitus: a randomised proof-of-concept study. Lancet 2001;357:331-5.

12 Cefalu WT, Skyler JS, Kourides IA et al. Inhaled human insulin treatment of patients with type 2 diabetes mellitus. Ann Intern Med 2001;134:203-7.

13 Cappelleri JC, Gerber RA, Kourides IA et al. Development and factor analysis of a questionnaire to measure patients' satisfaction with injected and inhaled insulin for type 1 diabetes. Diabetes Care 2000;12:1799-803.

14 The Veterans Affairs High-Density Lipoprotein Cholesterol Intervention Trial Study Group. Gemfibrozil for the secondary prevention of coronary heart disease in men with low levels of high-density lipoprotein cholesterol. N Engl J Med 1999;341:410-18.

15 Minhas R. Current progress in lipid therapy. Br J Cardiol 2003;10:59-68.

16 Olsson AG, Pears J, McKellar et al. Effect of rosuvastatin on low density lipoprotein cholesterol in patients with hypercholesterolaemia. Am J Cardiol 2001;88:504-8.

17 Davidson M, Ma P, Stein EA et al. Comparison of effects of low density lipoprotein cholesterol and high density lipoprotein cholesterol with rosuvastatin versus atorvastatin with type 11a or 11b hypercholesterolaemia. Am J Cardiol 2002;89:268-75.

18 Paoletti R, Fahmy M, Mahla G et al. ZD4522 is superior to pravastain and simvastatin in reducing LDL cholesterol, enabling more hypercholesterolaemic patients to achieve target LDL guidelines. J Am Coll Cardiol 2001;37(Suppl):291A abs 174.

19 Farnier M. Ezetimibe in hypercholesterolaemia. Int J Clin Prac. 2002;56:8.

20 Bays HE, Moore PB, Drehobl MA et al. Effectiveness and tolerability of ezetimibe in patients with primary hypercholesterolemia: pooled analysis of two phase II studies. Clin Ther 2001;23:1209-30.

21 Knopp RH, Gitter H, Truitt T et al. Ezetimibe reduces low density lipoprotein cholesterol: results of a phase III randomised, double-blind, placebo-controlled trial. Atherosclerosis 2001;2(suppl 2):38.Abstract.

22 Dujovne CA, Ettinger MP, McNeer JF et al. Ezetimibe, a selective cholesterol absorption inhibitor, improves plasma lipids in hypercholesterolemic patients. Circulation 2001;104(suppl II):176. Abstract.

23 Gagné C, Gaudet D, Bruckert E, for the Ezetimibe Study Group. Circulation 2002;105:2469-75.

24 Davidson M, McGarry T, Bettis R et al, for the Ezetimibe Study Group. Ezetimibe coadministered with simvastatin in 668 patients with primary hypercholesterolemia. J Am Coll Cardiol 2002;39(suppl A):226A.Abstract.

25 Ballantyne C, Houri J, Notarbartolo A et al, for the Ezetimibe Study Group. Ezetimibe coadministered with atorvastatin in 628 patients with primary hypercholesterolemia. J Am Coll Cardiol 2002;39(suppl A):227A. Abstract.

26 Stein E, Stender S, Mata P et al. Coadministration of ezetimibe plus atorvastatin. Atherosclerosis 2002;Suppl 3:211. Abstract.

27 Kosoglou T, Guillaume M, Sun S et al. Pharmacodynamic interaction between fenofibrate and the cholesterol absorption inhibitor ezetimibe. Atherosclerosis 2001;Suppl 2:38.Abstract.

28 Barnett AH. Pharmacology of antihypertensive drugs. In Barnett AH, Dodson PM (eds). Hypertension and Diabetes (third edition). London: Science Press Ltd, 2000 pp33-42.

129 Füsgen I, Schütz D. Use of indapamide SR in elderly patients in general practice. Results of a prospective study of 3,034 elderly multimorbid patients. Euro J Ger 2001;3(4):196-200.

130 Emeriau JP, Knauf H, Pujadas JO et al. A comparison of indapamide SR 1.5mg with both amlodipine 5mg and hydrochlorothiazide 25mg in elderly hypertensive patients: a randomised double-blind controlled study. J Hypertens 2001;19:343-50.

131 Leonetti G, Emeriau JP, Knauf H et al. Evaluation of long-term efficacy of indapamide SR 1.5mg in elderly hypertensive patients. Am J Hypertens 2001;14;4(Suppl 1):A102-A103.

132 Gosse P, Sheridan D, Zannad F et al. Left ventricular hypertrophy regression: Indapamide SR 1.5mg Versus Enalapril 20 mg (LIVE) study. J Hypertens 2000;18:1465-75.

133 Mallion J-M, Asmar R et al. Trough-to-peak ratio of indapamide 1.5mg sustained-release coated tablets assessed by ambulatory blood pressure monitoring. Archives des Maladies du Coeur et des Vaisseaux 1996; Special issue:2012.

134 Jaillon P, Asmar R, and the investigators of the 32-h ABPM Study. Thirty-two hour ambulatory blood pressure monitoring for the assessment of blood pressure evaluation in case of a missed dose of indapamide SR 1.5mg. European Society of Hypertension, Milan, 2001; Abstract.

135 PROGRESS Collaborative Group. Randomised trial of a perindopril-based blood pressure lowering regimen among 6105 individuals with previous stroke or transient ischaemic attack. Lancet 2001;358:1033-41.

136 ALLHAT Collaborative Research Group. Major outcomes in high risk, hypertensive, patients randomised to angiotensin converting enzyme inhibitor or calcium channel blocker versus diuretic. J Am Med Assoc 2002;288:2981-97.

137 Davis BR, Cutler JA, Gordon DJ et al. Rationale and design for the Antihypertensive and Lipid Lowering Treatmen to Prevent Heart Attack Trial (ALLHAT). ALL-HAT Research Group. Am J Hypertens 1996;9:342-60.

138 Brown JJ, Casals-Stenzel J, Cumming AMM et al. Angiotensin II, aldosterone and arterial pressure: a quantitative approach. Hypertension 1979;1:159-79.

139 Timmermans PBMWM. The discovery and physiological effects of a new class of highly specific angiotensin-II receptor antagonists. In Laragh JH, Brenner BN (eds). Hypertension Pathophysiology, Diagnosis and Management. New York: Raven Press, 1999;2351-60.

140 Mackenzie HS, Provoost AP, Troy JL et al. Antihypertensive and renal protective effects of irbesartan in fawn-hooded hypertensive rats. J Hypertens 1996, 14 (suppl. 1):S42.

141 Pohl M, Cooper M, Ulrey J et al. Safety and efficacy of irbesartan in hypertensive patients with type II diabetes and proteinuria. Am J Hypertens 1997;10:105A.

142 Parving H-H, Lehnert H, Brochner-Mortensen J et al. The effect of irbesartan on the development of diabetic nephropathy in patients with type 2 diabetes. N Engl J Med 2001;345:870-8.

143 Lewis EJ, Hunsicker LG, Clarke WR et al. Renoprotective effect of the angiotensin-receptor antagonist irbesartan in patients with nephropathy due to type 2 diabetes. N Engl J Med 2001;345:851-60.

144 Brenner BM, Cooper ME, de Zeeuw D et al. Effect of losartan on renal and cardiovascular outcomes in patients with type 2 diabetes and nephropathy. N Engl J Med 2001;345:861-9.

145 Dahlof B, Devereux RB, Kjeldsen SE et al. Cardiovascular morbidity and mortality in the Losartan Intervention For Endpoint reduction in hypertension study (LIFE): a randomised trial against atenolol. Lancet 2002;359:995-1010.

146 Dahlof B. Effects of angiotensin II blockade on cardiac hypertrophy and remodelling: a review. J Hum Hypertens 1995;9 (Suppl 5):37-44.

147 Colhoun HM, Dong W, Poulter NR. Blood pressure screening management and control in England: results from the health survey for England 1994. J Hypertens 1998;16:747-52.

148 Mogensen CE. Intervention strategies for microalbuminuria: the role of angiotensin II antagonists, including dual blockade with ACE-I and a receptor blocker (Abstract). Third International Symposium on Angiotensin II Antagonism, London, UK. 2000;A7.4.

149 Ysuf S. Two decades of progress in preventing vascular disease. Lancet 2002;360:2-3.

150 National service framework for diabetes. London: Department of Health, 2003

151 Hanif MW, Jones AF, Kumar S et al. Ethnic differences in risk factors for coronary heart disease in type 2 diabetes. Diabet Med 2002;19(Suppl 2):33 (Abstract).

152. Tuomilehto J, LindstromJ, Erikkson JG et al. Prevention of Type 2 Diabetes by changes in lifestyle among subjects with impaired glucose tolerance.N Engl J Med 2001; 344; 1343-50.

153. Jarrett RJ, Keen H, Fuller JH et al. Worsening to diabetes in men with impaired glucose tolerance. Diabetologia 1979;16; 25-30.

154. Pan XR, Li GW, Hu YH, Wang JX, Yang WY, An ZX et al. Effects of diet and exercise in preventing NIDDM in people with impaired glucose tolerance. The Da Qing IGT and Diabetes Study. Diabetes Care 1997;20:537-44.

155. DECODE Study Group on behalf of the European Epidemiology Study Group. Will new diagnostic criteria for diabetes mellitus change phenotype of patients with diabetes? Reanalysis of European epidemological data. Br Med J 1998; 317: 371-5.

156. DECODE Study Group. Age and sex specific prevalence of diabetes and impaired glucose regulation in 10 Asian cohorts. Diabetes Res Clin Prac 2002; 56: 540.

Index

Note: As the subject of this book is diabetes all entries refer to diabetes unless otherwise stated. Page numbers in italics refer to figures and/or tables. Abbreviations used in this index are the same as those listed on pages 105–106.

115